AF694567

Essentials of BLOOD BANKING

Essentials of BLOOD BANKING

A Handbook for
Students of Blood Banking and Clinical Residents

Second Edition

SR Mehdi MD
Professor of Hematology
Department of Pathology
Era's Lucknow Medical College
Lucknow, Uttar Pradesh, India

JAYPEE BROTHERS MEDICAL PUBLISHERS (P) LTD
New Delhi • London • Philadelphia • Panama

Jaypee Brothers Medical Publishers (P) Ltd.

Headquarters
Jaypee Brothers Medical Publishers (P) Ltd.
4838/24, Ansari Road, Daryaganj
New Delhi 110 002, India
Phone: +91-11-43574357
Fax: +91-11-43574314
Email: jaypee@jaypeebrothers.com

Overseas Offices
J.P. Medical Ltd.
83, Victoria Street, London
SW1H 0HW (UK)
Phone: +44-2031708910
Fax: +02-03-0086180
Email: info@jpmedpub.com

Jaypee-Highlights Medical Publishers Inc.
City of Knowledge, Bld. 237, Clayton
Panama City, Panama
Phone: +507-301-0496
Fax: +507-301-0499
Email: cservice@jphmedical.com

Jaypee Medical Inc.
The Bourse
111, South Independence Mall East
Suite 835, Philadelphia, PA 19106, USA
Phone: + 267-519-9789
Email: joe.rusko@jaypeebrothers.com

Jaypee Brothers Medical Publishers (P) Ltd.
17/1-B, Babar Road, Block-B, Shaymali
Mohammadpur, Dhaka-1207
Bangladesh
Mobile: +08801912003485
Email: jaypeedhaka@gmail.com

Jaypee Brothers Medical Publishers (P) Ltd.
Shorakhute, Kathmandu
Nepal
Phone: +00977-9841528578
Email: jaypee.nepal@gmail.com

Website: www.jaypeebrothers.com
Website: www.jaypeedigital.com

Inquiries for bulk sales may be solicited at: jaypee@jaypeebrothers.com

Essentials of Blood Banking

First Edition: 2006

Second Edition: **2013**

ISBN: 978-93-80704-52-4

Printed at Rajkamal Electric Press, Plot No. 2, Phase-IV, Kundli, Haryana.

Dedicated to

My parents

Preface to the Second Edition

Blood banking has come of age. The transfusion medicine is one of the thrust areas of medical research. The scare of transfusion-transmitted diseases and globalisation of AIDS have led to extraordinary media attention. The medicolegal aspects of blood banking act as a booster for maintaining quality and ensuring safety of blood.

Majority of the blood banks in the developing countries have developed their component laboratories. The use of whole blood is minimised day-by-day.

Almost all the departments of the hospital, surgical or non-surgical, hospital staff, medical or paramedical, and people in the form of patients or healthy blood donors come in contact of blood banks. The dissemination of knowledge of blood banking has become need of the hour.

I thank all my readers who had shown very good response to the first edition of this book.

Now, it is a pleasant feeling to write the preface for the second edition of the title *Essentials of Blood Banking (A Handbook for Students of Blood Banking and Clinical Residents)*. I have tried to incorporate in this edition the advancement in blood grouping and cross-matching techniques by the microtube gel method, screening of alloantibodies and apheresis. A new chapter on Obstetrical Transfusion Practice has also been added.

Many textbooks and technical manuals of blood banking are available in the market, but they are too exhaustive for the students who are not specialising in transfusion medicine and are interested only in the basic technical and clinical aspects of blood banking.

I hope this title would appeal to those students who look for a book on blood banking which is informative as well as handy.

I would like to thank my wife, daughter and son for providing me encouragement at each and every step of writing of the book. I am also indebted to my teachers and seniors who had always been a source of inspiration for me. I wish to thank my colleagues and students of medical colleges of Aligarh Muslim University, Aligarh, Uttar Pradesh, India, and King Saud University, Riyadh, Saudi Arabia, for creating an excellent academic and professional environment.

Last but not least, I thank M/s Jaypee Brothers Medical Publishers (P) Ltd, New Delhi, India, for advising me at each and every step of publication and coming out with the second edition of my title *Essentials of Blood Banking*.

SR Mehdi

Preface to the First Edition

In the last two decades, the progress in the field of blood banking has been phenomenal. Blood banking has grown up as transfusion medicine, an independent discipline. Blood banking is no more confined to only cross-matching and supply of blood. The spectrum of tests for transfusion-transmitted diseases is getting wider day-by-day. Pre-transfusion testing of blood for HIV1, HIV2, anti-HCV and in some of the countries, for HTLV1 has become mandatory, besides other tests. Newer techniques and latest generation testing kits are pouring in. Professional blood donors are banned.

HIV/AIDS awareness has shifted the focus of media on blood banks. Medicolegalities and ethical issues are very much in consideration. The talk of the day is Safety of the Blood. Regional transfusion centres have come up. Blood banks are directly under the supervision of the national and states AIDS Control Organisations.

The concept of whole blood transfusion has become obsolete. Transfusion of specific component of the blood has specific indications. A component laboratory is a must for every blood bank. The clinicians must be exposed to the usage and benefits of component therapy.

In this scenario, no person working in a hospital set-up, whether as a doctor or paramedic, can afford to be ignorant about the essentials of blood banking. The staff working in the transfusion services as "provider" and the clinicians and nurses acting as "facilitator" must ensure the transfusion of safe and disease-free blood to the "end user", i.e. the patient.

Therapeutic apheresis and stem cell collection have brought blood banking into clinical fold. Institutes are awarding MD and fellowships, exclusively in transfusion medicine. The progress and scope in the field of transfusion medicine is tremendous.

The handbook *Essentials of Blood Banking* deals with the basics of blood banking in brief, keeping in mind the requirements of the blood bank staff and the clinical residents. The blood bank personnel can refer to this book for techniques and the residents can carry the handbook to the wards. Even if one patient is saved of the complications of blood transfusion by the reader, the book will serve its purpose.

I wish to thank all my colleagues at the transfusion services of the Jawaharlal Nehru Medical College, Aligarh Muslim University, Aligarh, Uttar Pradesh, India, and the King Fahad Specialist Hospital, Buraidah, Kingdom of Saudi Arabia, who helped me to pick up the techniques of the trade by creating an enlightened and congenial working atmosphere. I would also like to thank National AIDS Control Organisation (NACO) and Uttar Pradesh State AIDS Control Society (UPSACS) for the best of the trainings and providing me an opportunity to serve as the Coordinator for Training of Trainers (TOT) Programme for HIV/AIDS.

SR Mehdi

Contents

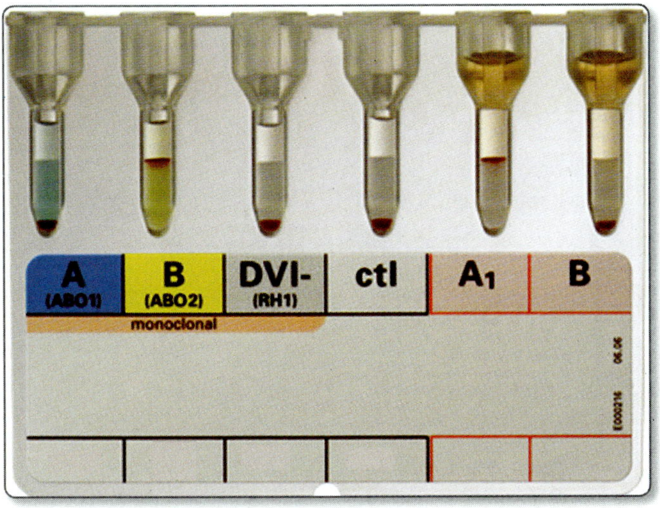

Figure 2.1: Gel card for ABO/D + Reverse grouping

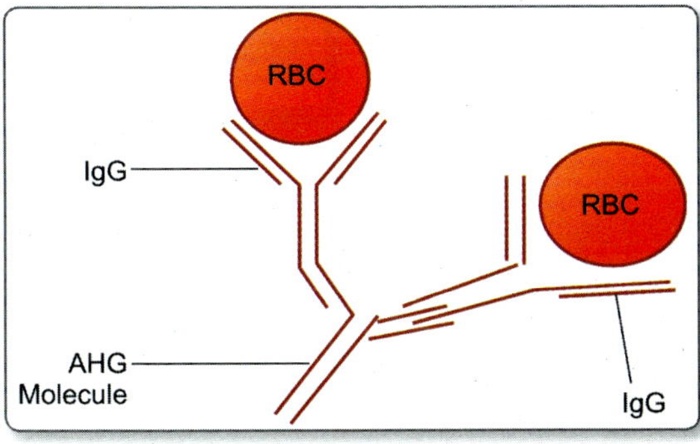

Figure 5.1: AHG molecule showing agglutination of RBC

Plate 2

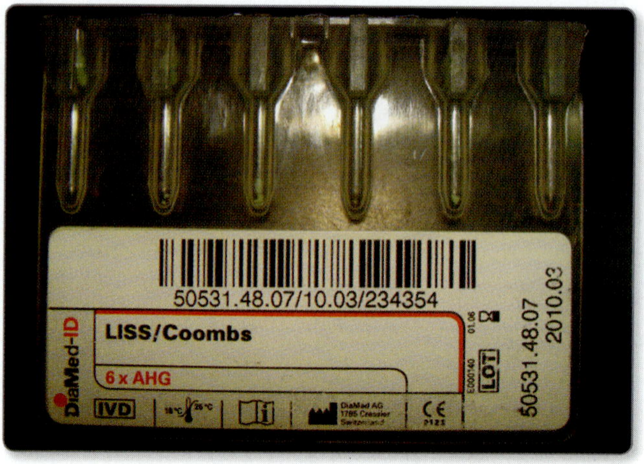

Figure 5.2: Gel card for DAT and IAT (Coombs' tests)

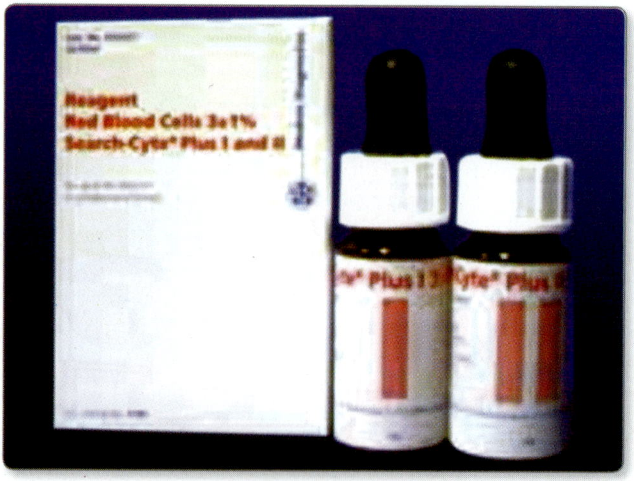

Figure 6.1: Two donor's primary panel of cells

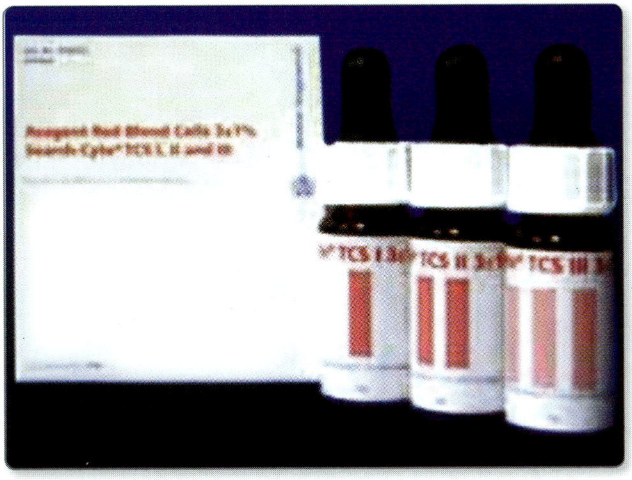

Figure 6.2: Three donor's primary panel of cells

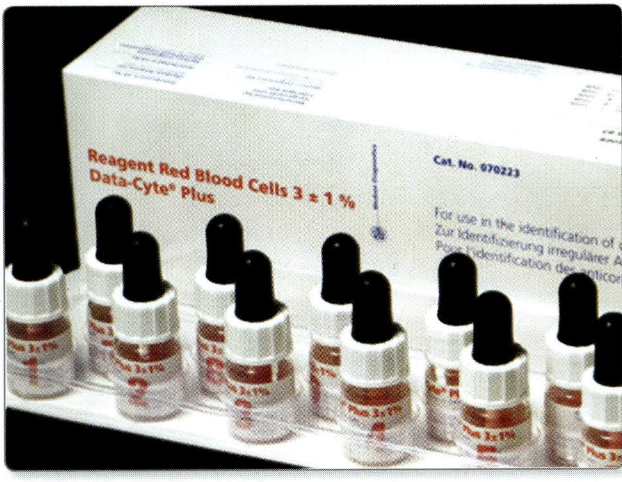

Figure 6.3: Secondary panel of antibodies screening cells

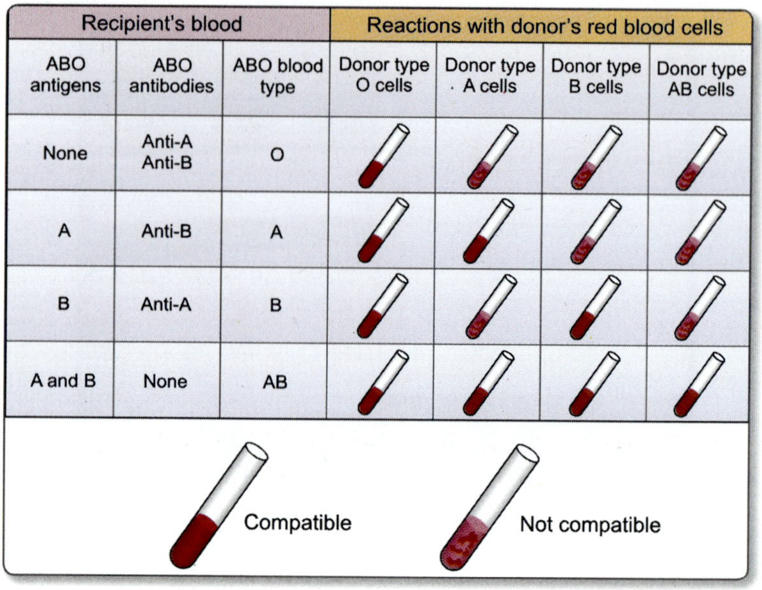

Figure 7.1: Diagrammatic presentation of ABO compatibility

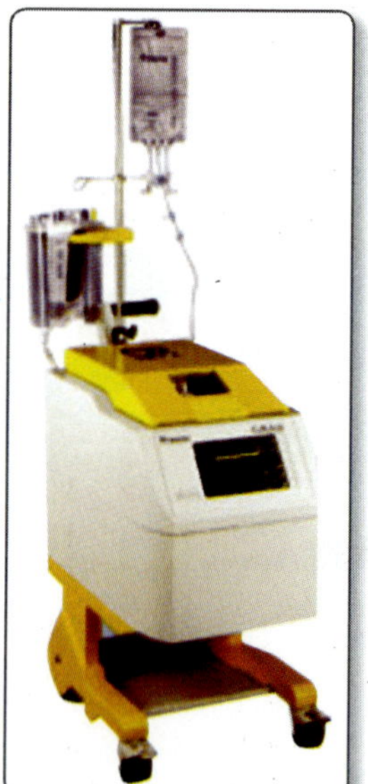

Figure 15.1 Intraoperative blood salvage machine (Cell Saver)

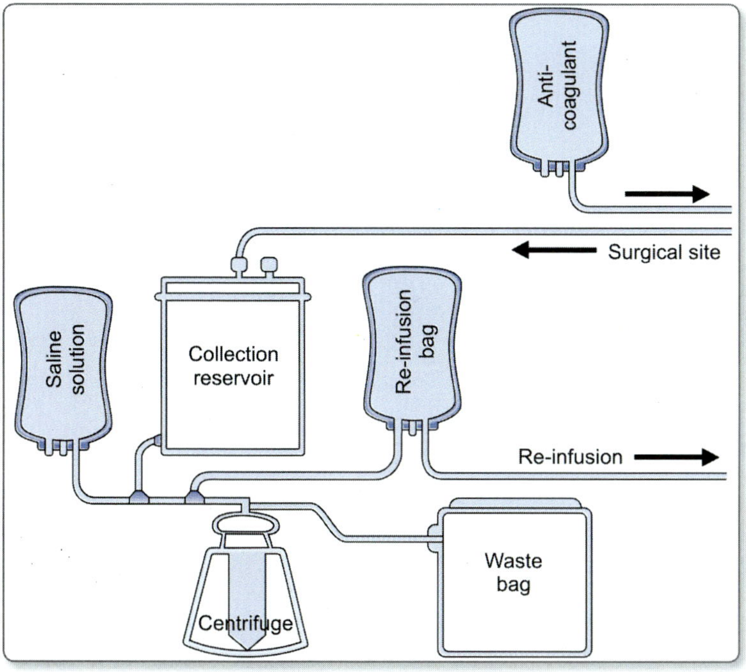

Figure 15.2: Intraoperative blood salvage diagram

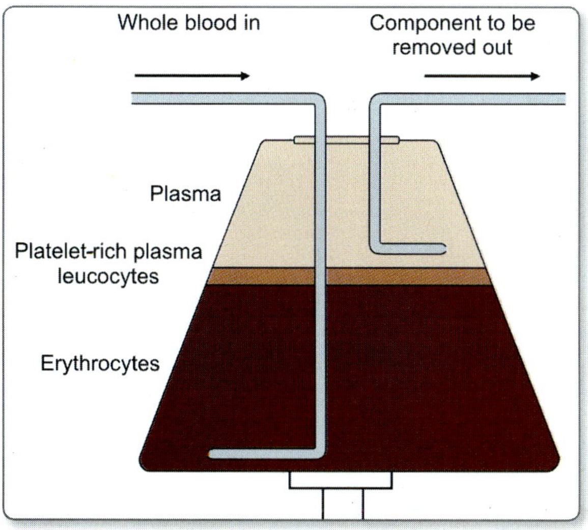

Figure 15.3: Diagrammatic presentation of functioning of apheresis

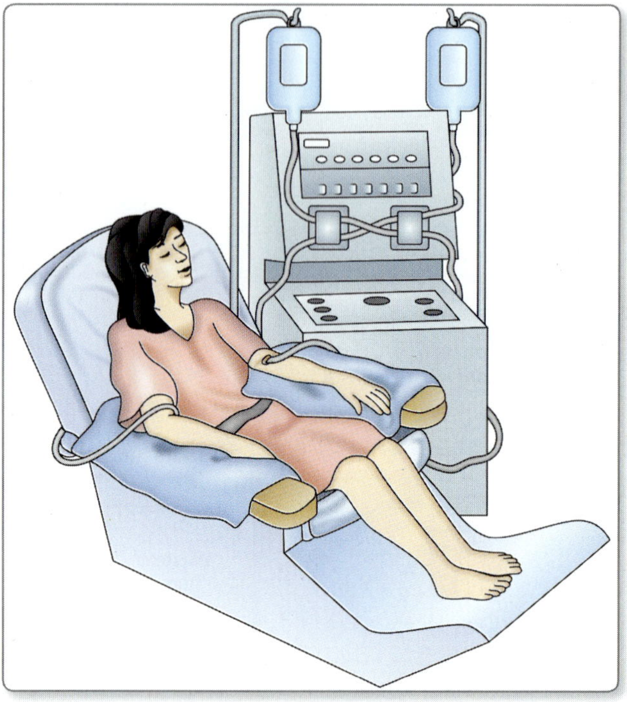

Figure 15.4: Functioning of a continuous flow separator

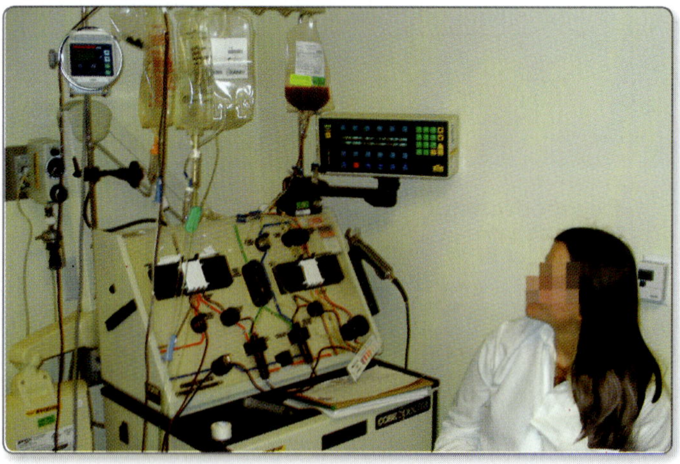

Figure 15.5: Therapeutic apheresis in progress

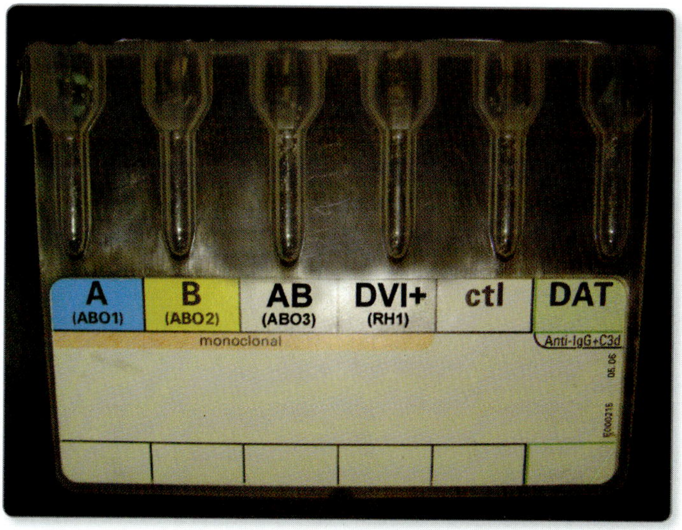

Figure 16.1: ABO blood grouping for newborns and DAT

chapter 1

Immunohaematology

The immune system has evolved as a highly specialised function of human beings, which is concerned with the substances considered "foreign" to the body. It consists of a cellular component and a humoral component. Although the field of blood group serology is associated mainly with the humoral component of the immune system, the mechanics of antibody production in vivo involves the cellular arm of the immune system or the cell-mediated immunity.

The science of immunohaematology deals with the basic principles of antigen and antibody structure, the genetics, the biochemistry, its mode of action and its role in haematology. To understand the principle of compatibility testing and transfusion reactions the basic knowledge of immunohaematology is essential.

Antigen

Antigen is a substance, which elicits immune response. It is a complex molecule whose molecular weight exceeds 10000 daltons. The ABH antigens are glycolipids while Rh antigens are protein. The hepatitis B surface antigen (HbsAg) is a lipoprotein.

A number of characteristics influence the antigenicity. These include the molecular size, charge on the surface of cells and the solubility. The inheritance of Ir genes and occurrence of disease also influence the antibody response.

Not all the blood group substances are equally immunogenic. Approximately 50% of Rh-negative recipients of Rh-positive blood have the tendency to get sensitised to the D antigen. Other Rh antigens like C and E and antigens of other blood group systems are relatively less immunogenic. The number of antigen sites on the RBC varies according to specificity. There are approximately 1 million ABO antigen sites and 25000 Rh (D) antigen sites on a RBC.

Antibody

The antibodies are immunoglobulin in nature. Approximately 82-96% of antibodies are polypeptide, and the rest 4-18% are carbohydrates in nature.

Production

The antibodies are produced in the plasma of those individuals who lack the corresponding antigen. The production may be because of either blood transfusion or foetomaternal leak of incompatible blood.

Immunoglobulin structure

All the immunoglobulins share a common chemical structural configuration. Each basic antibody unit is composed of *four* polypeptide chains: *two* identical *light chains* having a molecular weight (M.W) of approximately 22500 daltons and *two* identical heavy chains with a M.W of 50000-75000 daltons. Covalent disulfide bonds hold the four chains together. Each heavy chain has 440 amino acids and each light chain 220 amino acids.

The chemical structure of heavy chains is responsible for the diversity of immunoglobulin classes. The light chains *kappa* and *lambda* are common to all immunoglobulins.

Immunoglobulin classes

The isotypes of the heavy chains determine the class of immuno-globulin. There are five classes of immunoglobulins designated as IgA, IgD, IgE, IgG and IgM.

The blood group antibodies are commonly, IgM, IgG or IgA.

IgA

IgA class of antibodies exists both as a monomer and as polymers. The M.W is approximately 160000 daltons.

IgG

The IgG constitutes approximately 75% of total serum immuno-globulins. It is a Y-shaped monomer. There are four subclasses of IgG; IgG1, IgG2, IgG3 and IgG4 based on the sequence of amino acids in the heavy chain.

The IgG antibodies react at 37°C.

The MW of IgG is 150000 daltons which is the lowest of all immunoglobulins. It enables IgG to cross the placental barrier.

IgM

The IgM antibodies constitute approximately 10% of the total serum immunoglobulins. They are pentamer in shape. The M.W is 900000 daltons which makes it the heaviest of all classes of immunoglobulins. It does not cross the placental barrier.

They react at room temperature (20-24°C).

The IgM are highly effective agglutinins and are capable of activating the complement. Plasma contains significant amounts of IgM.

Complete and incomplete antibodies

The antibodies, which are produced without any antigenic stimulus, are known as complete antibodies. Most IgM class antibodies fall in this category. They are capable of agglutinating red cells suspended in normal saline at 20-25°C. Most of the ABH antibodies are IgM in nature, and called *natural or complete* antibodies.

The antibodies that require a bridge like the Coomb's molecule for binding to the antigenic site are called incomplete antibodies. Most IgG antibodies are incomplete antibodies. They react at 37°C. The Rh (CDE) are *incomplete* or *acquired* antibodies.

Monoclonal and polyclonal antibodies

The antibodies, which are derived from multiple ancestral clones of antibody producing cells and carry both *kappa* and *lambda* light chains are termed as *polyclonal antibodies*. In contrast, the antibodies, which contain exclusively *kappa* or *lambda* light chains, are known as *monoclonal antibodies.* Monoclonal antibodies have the ability to recognise single antigenic epitope, and provide greater diagnostic precision than polyclonal antibodies.

Identification and estimation of immunoglobulin

The specificity of the blood group antibodies is determined by two methods. Either by 2-mercaptoethanol treatment or by separating the antibody on column chromatography. The haemagglutination inhibition technique is applied for estimation of IgG, IgM and IgA class of antibodies.

Antigen antibody ratio

The speed by which antigen and antibody bind, is dependent on number of antibody molecules in the medium and the antigen sites available on the cell. By raising the serum to cell ratio the number of molecules are increased. If 2 drops of cell suspension are added to 4 drops of serum that increases the sensitivity of the test. The other factors affecting the binding of antigen antibody are pH of the medium, temperature and incubation period.

Complement

The complements are plasma proteins that interact with bound antibodies resulting in cell lysis and enhanced phagocytosis.

The nine components of complements are designated from C1 to C9. The C4 acts in between 1 and 2, the rest being in numerical order.

The complements are destroyed when heated with anticoagulants to 56°C for 30 minutes.

Sensitisation

The sensitisation is defined as binding of antigen and antibody, in *vitro* or *in vivo*, with or without agglutination.

Agglutination

Whenever the sensitised cells come into contact of each other, the result is clumping of red cells known as agglutination.

Grades of agglutination

The agglutination results are graded from 1+ to 4+. The American Association of Blood Banks (AABB) recommends the following grading system:

4+ = One solid aggregate of red cells
3+ = Several large aggregates
2+ = Medium sized aggregates with a clear background
1+ = Small aggregates with a turbid background giving granular appearance.
Weak (w) = Tiny aggregates are seen only under microscope
Negative = All cells are free.

Factors influencing agglutination

The following factors affect the process of agglutination.

Charge on cells

The red cells carry negative charge on their surface and repel each other, but when the Na+ present in the normal saline medium is added the negative charge is reduced, ultimately reducing the total charge, called zeta potential.

Albumin or enzymes

The type of the medium used affects the agglutination. The bovine albumin or enzyme papain reduces further the zeta potential. The IgG molecules form bridges between red cells, resulting in agglutination.

Effect of Coomb's serum

The Coomb's or antihuman globulin molecule (AHG) forms bridge between different molecules of IgG immunoglobulin and approximates the sensitised cells leading to agglutination.

Haemolysis

The antigen and antibody reaction where complement is activated leading to breakdown of red cells and release of haemoglobin is called haemolysis.

ABO blood group system

chapter 2

Karl Landsteiner opened the doors of blood banking with his discovery of first blood group system; ABO, in the year 1901. The blood groups were divided in A, B, AB and O.

The nomenclature of different blood groups is based on the presence or absence of particular *antigen* on the surface of red cells.

Inheritance of ABO blood groups

Bernstein first described the theory of inheritance of ABO blood groups in 1924. He demonstrated that each individual inherits one ABO gene from each parent and the presence of these two genes determines the type of antigen present on the surface of red cells. The gene A, B or O occupy one locus on each chromosome 9.

Genotypes and Phenotypes

The genotypes and phenotypes of ABO group are listed in Table 2.1.

Antigens of ABO groups

A and B genes do not produce antigens directly, but produce enzymes called glycosyl transferases which add specific sugars to oligosaccharide chains and are converted to H substance by the action of H gene.

The expression of A and B genes is dependent on H gene.

The H gene is converted to H substance. Subsequently, the H substance is acted upon by specific transferases and is converted to either A or B antigen. Some H substance remains unconverted and is

Table 2.1: Genotypes and phenotypes of ABO group

Group	Genotype	Phenotype
A	AA	A
	AO	
B	BB	B
	BO	
O	OO	O

expressed as H antigen. There is no conversion of H substance to either antigen A or B in O blood group. Hence, the maximum amount of H antigen is found on O red cells.

The H antigen is present on the red cells in the following diminishing quantity.

$O > A_2 > B > A_2B > A_1 > A_1B$

The ABO antigens are found on all the cells of the body tissues. The ABO compatibility is a prerequisite in cases of organ transplants.

ABO antibodies

ABO antibodies are generally IgM in nature. They are naturally occurring, complete and cold reacting antibodies, which do not cross placental barrier, and are capable of binding the complement.

If the antigen is missing in a blood group, the corresponding antibody is present.

The following antigens and antibodies are present in ABO system (Table 2.2).

The anti-AB of O blood group carries a higher titre than anti-A or anti-B.

The anti-A and anti-B present in O blood group are more often IgG in nature and are known as haemolysins.

Antibodies in infants

The IgM anti-A and anti-B are not produced up to the age of 3 to 6 months. The maximum titre reaches by the age of 5 to 10 years.

Whatever antibodies are present in a newborn are of maternal origin.

ABO subgroups

The subgroups of A and AB are of clinical significance.

Table 2.2: ABO group antigens and antibodies

ABO Group	Antigen	Antibodies
A	A and H	anti-B
B	B and H	anti-A
AB	A, B and H	NONE
O	H	anti-A, anti-B and occasionally anti-AB

Subgroups of A

The group A has been subclassified in A_1 and A_2 depending on their reaction to antisera anti-A and anti-A_1.

A_1

The A red cells which react with both anti-A and anti-A_1 are designated as A_1 subgroup. The A_1 has more antigenic sites for A antigen and less for H. The antibody present in A_1 is only anti-B.

A_2

The A red cells which react with only anti-A and not with anti-A_1 are called A_2. This is a weak A subgroup and carries more H substance. In 1-8% of cases of A_2 subgroup, anti-A_1 is also present beside anti-B.

The cells of approximately 80% of A individuals are A_1, while the remaining 20% are A_2.

The other weak and clinically not significant A subgroups are A_3, Ax and Am.

Subgroups of AB

Like A the AB is also subclassified in A_1B and A_2B subgroups. The A_1B cells carry minimum amount of H antigen. Approximately, 22-35% of A_2B individuals produce anti-A_1 antibodies.

The anti-A_1 present in A_2 or A_2B individuals is usually a cold reactive clinically insignificant antibody, unless it reacts at 37°C.

Bombay blood group (Oh phenotype)

The O blood group individuals do not carry either A or B antigen, but have maximum amount of H antigen on their red cells. Some individuals lack even H antigen along with A and B. These individuals are called Oh phenotype. Since there is no H antigen on the surface of red cells of Oh, the anti-H antibody develops in their serum, along with all the other antibodies found in any O blood group. The anti-H present in Oh is clinically significant, warm antibody reactive at 37°C.

Bhende YM, et al in year 1952, first discovered this blood group in the city of Bombay, India, from where it got its name.

The Bombay blood group is not compatible with any ABO blood group, and the choice of blood for these individuals remains only Bombay itself.

Antisera used in ABO grouping

The following commercially prepared antisera are used in detection of ABO blood groups:

Antisera A

The "Methylene Blue" dye present in antisera A gives it a blue colour. Antisera A carry very high titres of anti-A antibodies.

Antisera B

The presence of dye "Acriflavin" in antisera B gives it a yellow colour. The antisera B is rich in anti-B antibodies.

Antisera AB

The antisera AB is colourless, which is used for detection of weak A and B antigens.

ABO grouping

The ABO grouping can be performed by the following two methods:

- Slide method
- Spin tube method.

Slide method

This is a simple technique, which should be employed in cases of emergency or outdoor camps. The technique is less sensitive and not capable of detecting weak antigens.

Procedure

1. The test can be performed either on glass slides or on ceramic tiles.
2. Place one drop of anti-A and one drop of anti-B sera on two previously labelled slides.
3. Add one drop of blood (preferably 20% red cell suspension) on each slide.
4. Mix properly by a clean glass stick or the corner of another slide.
5. Rock the slides in order to mix the cells and sera and leave at room temperature for 2 minutes.
6. Record the results.

Table 2.3: Interpretation of results of ABO grouping

Anti-A	Anti-B	Blood group
+	–	A
–	+	B
+	+	AB
–	–	O

Interpretation of results

The agglutination appears like granular precipitate resembling yogurt. Agglutination (+) in one or both antisera is interpreted as follows (Table 2.3):

Tube method

This is a more sensitive technique which is capable of detecting weak antigens and antibodies. The cell grouping and serum groupings are performed separately, and are complimentary to each other.

Washing of red cells

Before going for any procedure in the blood bank, the red cells have to be washed properly. 0.5 ml of red cells are mixed with normal saline filling 2/3rd of test tube. The mixture is centrifuged at 3000 rpm for 1 minute. The supernatant is discarded. Refill the tube with same amount of normal saline and centrifuge again. Repeat the procedure three times and discard the supernatant every time. The remaining cells are washed cells.

Preparation of 5% red cell suspension

Mix the washed red cells and the normal saline in one of the following ratios as per requirement:
0.1 ml of cells + 1.9 ml of normal saline
0.2 ml of cells + 3.8 ml of normal saline
0.5 ml of cells + 9.5 ml of normal saline
Centrifuge the mixture at 1000 rpm for 1 minute.

Procedure

Cell grouping (forward grouping) (Table 2.4)

1. Prepare 5% red cell suspension (tomato colour) in normal saline.
2. Add 1 drop of anti-A in the tube labelled A, anti-B in the tube labeled B and anti-AB in the tube labelled AB.

Table 2.4: Interpretation of results of ABO forward and reverse grouping

Forward grouping			Reverse grouping			Blood group
Anti-A	Anti-B	Anti-AB	A	B	O	
+	+	+	–	–	–	AB
+	–	+	–	+/H	–	A
–	+	+	+/H	–	–	B
–	–	–	+/H	+/H	–	O

+ = Agglutination, – = No agglutination, H = Haemolysis
The Bombay blood group (Oh) phenotype serum would be showing agglutination even with O group cells on reverse grouping.

3. Add 1 drop of the cell suspension in each tube.
4. Mix properly, incubate the mixture at room temperature (RT) for 5-10 minutes and then centrifuge at 1000 rpm for 1 minute.
5. If no haemolysis is observed in the supernatant, disperse the cell button.
6. Check for agglutination. If no clump is seen by naked eyes, examine under microscope for weak agglutination.
7. Record the results.

Serum grouping (reverse grouping) (Table 2.4)

1. The serum of the donor/patient is tested against known cells of group A, B and O. These cells are either prepared in the lab by pooling or can be acquired from manufacturers.
2. Arrange three test tubes and label them A, B and O.
3. Place 2 drops of the serum to be tested in each tube.
4. Add 1 drop of A group cells to the tube A, B group cells to tube B and O group cells to the tube labelled O.
5. Shake the contents gently. Incubate at RT for 5-10 minutes and centrifuge at 1000 rpm for 1 minute.
6. If the supernatant shows no signs of haemolysis, disperse the cell button and observe for agglutination.
7. If no agglutination is observed by naked eyes, examine under microscope.
8. Record the results.

ABO gel grouping

The gel technique by its ID card system has made the blood grouping a very convenient procedure. Forward and reverse ABO grouping and Rh grouping are done with a single card in a very short time.

Reagents

The "ID-card ABO/D + reverse grouping for patients". The microtubes contain the following reagents **(Figure 2.1)**.

- Microtube 1 - anti-A
- Microtube 2 - anti-B
- Microtube 3 - anti-D
- Microtube 4 - negative Rh control
- Microtube 5 - A1 cells
- Microtube 6 - B cells.

Additional reagents required

- ID- diluent 2: It is modified LISS for red cell suspension
- Ready to use ID known cells A_1 and B, 0.8% suspension in 10 ml vials.

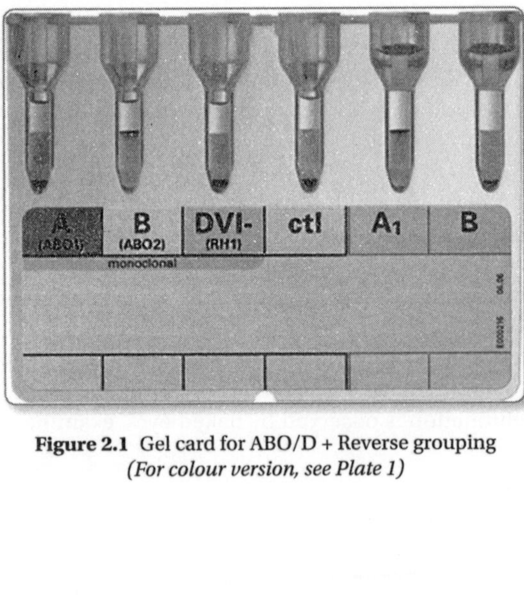

Figure 2.1 Gel card for ABO/D + Reverse grouping
(For colour version, see Plate 1)

Further materials required

- ID - Dispenser
- ID - Pipette
- ID - Tips
- Tubes for suspensions
- ID - Working table
- ID - Centrifuge

Sample required

Freshly drawn blood samples in EDTA or citrate.

For reverse grouping, either plasma or serum can be used.

Preparation of blood samples

Prepare 5% cell suspension.

- Bring the ID-diluent 2 at room temperature
- Dispense 0.5 ml of ID-diluent 2 into a clean tube
- Add 50 μL of whole blood or 25 μL of packed cells, mix gently.

Procedure

1. Write the patient or donor's name and registration number on the ID card.
2. Remove the aluminium foil from the top of the microtubes by holding the card in the upright position.
3. Pipette 10 μL of patient's 5% red cell suspension to the microtubes 1-4 (A, B, D and control (ctl)).
4. Place 50 μL of ID-cell A_1 in microtube 5 (A_1).
5. Place 50 μL ID-cell B in microtube 6 (B).
6. Centrifuge the ID card for 10 minutes in the ID-centrifuge.
7. Read and record the results.

Result

Positive

Agglutinated cells forming a red line on the surface of the gel.

Negative

Compact button of cells on the bottom of the microtube.

Interpretation of results

The result of the ID card is also interpreted as the results of the test tube method, considering the microtubes 1and 2 as forward grouping, 3 as Rh, 4 as negative Rh control, 5 and 6 as reverse grouping.

The negative control must not show any agglutination. If it shows agglutination, your procedure is invalid. Repeat the whole procedure.

Precautions

- ID cards which show air bubbles in the gel or drops in the upper part, or the covering aluminium foil is removed, the ID card must be discarded.
- Bacterial or other contamination of materials may cause false positive or false negative results.

ABO subgrouping

The clinically significant subgroups, which are detected in laboratory, are A_1, A_2, A_1B and A_2B.

The anti-A_1 can be obtained either from lectin seeds called Dolichos biflorus or from the human sera of A_2 individuals.

Procedure

1. Arrange two test tubes.
2. Place 2 drops of anti-A_1 reagent in the tube-1.
3. Place 2 drops of anti-A reagent in the tube-2.
4. Add 1 drop of 5% washed cells of A group to be tested, in each tube.
5. Mix the contents of each tube by shaking, incubate at RT for 5-10 minutes and centrifuge at 1000 rpm for 1 minute.
6. Disperse the cell button and examine for agglutination. All the negative results must be examined under microscope.
7. Record the results.

It is advisable to run parallel controls with known A_1 and A_2 cells. Interpretation of results of A subgrouping is given in Table 2.5.

Table 2.5: Interpretation of results of A subgrouping

Tube-1	Tube-2	Blood group
Anti- A_1	Anti-A	
+	+	A_1
–	+	A_2

+ = Agglutination, – = No agglutination

ABO discrepancies

If the results of forward and reverse grouping do not correspond with each other, the condition is known as ABO discrepancy. The ABO discrepancies are usually technical in nature. Before forming an opinion on the real ABO discrepancy, the following information about the patient must be collected.

- Patient's age
- Diagnosis
- Transfusion history
- Medications
- Immune status
- H/O pregnancy.

The common sources of error resulting in ABO discrepancies are listed below.

- Misidentification of blood samples or test tubes.
- Cell suspension either too heavy or too light.
- Failure to add reagent.
- A mix-up in samples.
- Clerical errors.
- Inaccurate centrifuge.
- Contaminated reagents.
- Failure to follow manufacturer's instructions.

Group I discrepancy

This is the commonest type of discrepancy. The discrepancy I occurs as a result of weak reacting, depressed or missing antibodies. In the following population, this discrepancy is seen more often.

- Newborns.
- Elderly patients.
- Patients of chronic lymphocytic leukaemia, prolymphocytic leukaemia and lymphomas. The probable cause of depressed antibodies in these conditions is hypogammaglobulinaemia.
- Patients of AIDS.
- Patients on immunosuppressive drugs.
- Post-bone marrow transplant.

Group II discrepancy

The discrepancy is between forward and reverse grouping, owing to weak or missing antigens. This is quite uncommon type of discrepancy. Some of the common causes in this group II discrepancy are:

- Subgroups may be present.

- Weak expression of A or B antigens in cases of leukaemias, or occasionally in Hodgkin's disease.
- *Acquired B antigen:* The forward grouping shows presence of A and B antigens and the group appears AB but the serum contains anti-B. A1 cells are notorious for such type of expression. This phenomenon is frequently encountered in patients of carcinoma colon and rectum.

Group III discrepancy

This discrepancy between forward and reverse grouping usually occurs due to abnormalities of plasma proteins. The common conditions resulting in type III discrepancy are:

- Multiple myeloma.
- Waldenstrom's macroglobulinaemia.
- Other plasma cell dyscrasias.

Group IV discrepancy

The discrepancy may be a result of miscellaneous problems. Some of the common causes are:

- *Polyagglutination:* Bacterial or viral contamination of blood causes exposure of a hidden erythrocyte antigen called "T antigen" which leads to spontaneous agglutination of red cells by most normal adult sera containing anti-T. A few characteristics of this reaction are.
- The red cells are agglutinated only by fresh adult serum and not by cord serum as the cord serum does not contain anti-T, anti-Tn and anti-Tk.
- Direct Coomb's Test (DCT) is negative.
- Agglutination is strongest at room temperature showing absence of cold agglutinins.
- *Unexpected alloantibodies:* The patient's serum reacting with other than A and B antigens, present on the surface of known cells, is used for reverse grouping.

Resolution of ABO discrepancies

Before proceeding further to resolve the discrepancy between forward and reverse grouping the discrepancy is to be established by ruling out all the common sources of error. The following steps are to be taken:

- Repeat all the tests on fresh samples.
- Wash the cells 3-4 times to rule out rouleaux formation.
- If the discrepancy persists in the repeat results, the following work up is to be performed.

Type I

- Reverse group reaction is to be enhanced.
- Incubate the patient's serum with the reagent cells at room temperature for 15 minutes.
- If no reaction is observed, incubate the mixture at 4°C and 37°C for 15-30 minutes to enhance the antigen-antibody reaction.
- Auto-control and an O cell control must be run concurrently.

Type II

- Acidify the anti-B typing reagent to pH 6.0. The acidified serum would agglutinate only "true B antigen" and not the "acquired B antigen".

Type III

- Differentiate between rouleaux formation and agglutination. Rouleaux formation can be dispersed by adding a drop of saline to the cell and serum mixture on the slide.
  The true agglutination would persist.
- In case Wharton's jelly causes rouleaux formation, the cells should be washed at least 8 times.

Type IV

The patient showing polyagglutinability should be transfused only washed red cells and not the plasma containing whole blood, since the plasma contains anti-T.

chapter 3

Rh blood group system

The Rh blood group system is a complex system, and certain aspects of its genetics and nomenclature are still unsettled.

The human antibody directed against the D antigen was first noticed in the serum of a group O woman who had a history of stillbirths and transfusion reactions. Levine and Stetson reported it in the year 1939.

In 1940, Landsteiner and Wiener raised an antibody from the serum of guinea pigs and rabbits by immunising them with the red cells of Rhesus monkey. The same antibody agglutinated the red cells of 85% of the human beings. The antibody was called anti-Rh, and its antigenic determinant Rh factor due to its similarities with the antigen found in the Rhesus (Rh) monkey.

Wiener and Peters in the year of 1940 isolated human anti-Rh antibody from the sera of individuals transfused with ABO compatible Rh positive blood. Further studies established that the animal anti-Rh and human anti-Rh are not identical, but by that time it was too late and Rh blood group system had received its name.

Nomenclature

The following three types of nomenclature have been postulated for Rh blood group system.

Rh-Hr terminology

Wiener proposed that gene product is a single entitity agglutinogen on the surface of red cells and each agglutinogen has number of antigens, recognised by its own specific antibody.

A capital R denotes the presence of the original factor in an agglutinogen, where as r as subscript indicates the lack of the factor. Rho represents D while rh' and rh" represent C and E.

DCE terminology

Fisher and Race in 1944 defined the antigens of the Rh system as D,C,E,c and e. The same letters were used for genes too, but the genes were written in italics. The corresponding antibodies of these antigens are anti-D, anti-C, anti-E, anti-c and anti-e. DCE is the easiest and widely accepted system of nomenclature.

The Fisher Race Rh gene combination is given in Table 3.1.

Table 3.1: Fisher Race Rh gene combinations

Fisher Race		Short notions
Gene complex	*Antigens*	
CDe	C,D,e	R_1
cDE	c.D.E	R_2
cDe	c,D.e	R_0
CDE	C,D,E	R_z
Cde	C, e	r
cde	c,e	r'
cdE	c,E	r"
CdE	C,E	R_y

Numerical terminology

Rosenfield and coworkers in 1960 proposed this system, which assigns a number to each antigen. The corresponding names of the systems of Fisher and Rosenfield are as follows:

D is Rh1
C is Rh2
E is Rh3
c is Rh4
e is Rh5.

The absence of an antigen is designated by a prefix as a negative sign, e.g. if c and e antigens are absent, the designation is:

Rh:1, 2, 3, –4, –5.

Inheritance

Wiener proposed theory of single gene producing single product that contained separate recognisable factors. Fisher postulated theory of three genes on Rh locus that controlled production of their respective genes.

The gene controlling D antigen resides on chromosome 1. It is autosomal dominant in character.

Biochemical structure of Rh antigens

There are different views regarding biochemical structure of Rh antigens, but one authentic opinion is, that they are proteins with phospholipid content. Rh haplotypes encode three distinct non-glycosylated polypeptide chains carrying D,Cc and Ee epitopes.

Unlike ABO antigens the Rh antigens are expressed only on erythrocytes and not on other body tissues including leucocytes and platelets.

Clinical significance

The D antigen is as significant in transfusion practice as A and B antigens. *The anti-D is not found in all D negative individuals.* The formation of anti-D is always, almost after exposure of a D negative person to D positive blood, either through transfusion or pregnancy. More than 80% of D negative persons develop anti-D after transfusion of a single unit of D positive blood.

Types of Rh antigens

The five commonly detected antigens are D, C, E, c and e, of which D is the most potent and highly immunogenic, followed by c and E. The commonly used terms of Rh+ (positive) and Rh – (negative) depends on the presence or absence of D antigen.

Approximately 95% of Indians are Rh positive while only 85% of Caucasians (whites) show Rh positivity.

The D weak or D^u phenotype

It has been observed that certain D positive red cells are not agglutinated by all anti-D sera, but require antihuman globulin (Coomb's) sera in indirect Coomb's test (ICT) to show agglutination. The phenomenon is nothing but a weak expression of the D antigen. This particular D phenotype is called D^U. So, D^U is not a different antigen but a differing expression of D antigen.

D^U transfusion policy

All D^U donor units are considered Rh positive and transfused only to Rh positive recipients.

Usually the recipients are not tested for D^U and are considered Rh negative, hence safely transfused Rh negative blood. In case of short supply of Rh negative blood the recipient should also be tested and if comes out D^U positive, may be transfused Rh positive blood.

If the mother carries anti-D antibody then the D^U infant is likely to suffer from haemolytic disease of newborn (HDN).

Rh null syndrome

The individuals lack not only D but all the Rh antigens. They have a type of haemolytic anaemia caused by an abnormal cell membrane. These individuals are more prone to develop anti-D antibody.

Rh antibodies

The Rh antibodies are clinically significant and are capable of causing haemolytic transfusion reaction (HTR). Most of the Rh antibodies and specially anti-D require antigenic stimulus to develop. The Rh antibodies result from immunisation by either transfusion or pregnancy. Only anti-C and anti-E can occur without known antigenic stimulus.

The Rh antibodies are mostly IgG, and react best in enzyme or antiglobulin medium, but anti-C has been detected in saline test indicating its IgM nature.

Generally, Rh antibodies do not bind complement.

Rh grouping reagents

The following types of anti-D sera are being used:

- *Low protein anti-D serum:* This is a typical saline reacting anti-D which is employed in tube tests. The two types available are:
  - Saline reagent prepared from raw material containing IgM, which reacts with antigens, suspended in saline without any potentiater.
  - Anti-D serum prepared from IgG antibodies which have been chemically modified to react in saline medium.
- *High protein anti-D sera:* These antisera contain macromolecular additives. It is advisable to use these sera with the control provided by the manufacturer.
- *Polyclonal anti-D sera:* These antisera require potentiators like albumin, enzymes or Coomb's (AHG) serum to react with IgG anti-D.
- *Monoclonal anti-D sera:* This antiserum is preferred and is commonly used because of its specificity and ability to react equally at 20°C and 37°C for slide and rapid tube tests.

The three types of monoclonal anti-D are:

- IgM anti-D monoclonal serum.
- IgM or IgG monoclonal anti-D serum.
- Blend of IgG anti-D polyclonal and IgM monoclonal.

The quality and suitability of anti-D reagent depends on the following:

- The reagent must have a suitable titre for albumin replacement technique. The titre should not be lower than 1:128.
- The reagent must be specific for the corresponding antigen being tested.

Tests for Rh grouping

In most of the blood banks the routine typing for Rh is carried out for D antigen only. The tests for other Rh antigens are recommended in specific conditions, such as finding compatible blood for a person showing an alloantibody in his serum or for paternity testing.

Techniques

The Rh testing is routinely done by saline method only, but at times, the potentiaters like albumin or enzyme (papain) or AHG serum may be required.

There are mainly two techniques for Rh grouping:

- Slide test
- Tube test.

Slide test

The technique is simple but not reliable. It is recommended for outdoor camps and not for routine testing in the blood banks. The weakly reactive cells may not give a positive test.

Procedure

1. Place 1 drop of anti-D reagent on the slide labelled test.
2. Place 1 drop of normal saline (no anti-D) on another slide.
3. Add 1 drop of whole blood, or 50% red cells suspended in plasma on both the slides.
4. Mix the cells and the reagent by a clean stick or corner of another slide and spread the mixture.
5. Rock the slide gently for 2 minutes.
6. Place both the slides on a glass view box, which is not only the light source but maintains approximately 37°C temperature at the bottom of the slide.
7. *Record the results:* Agglutination on the test slide and smooth suspension on the control is a positive test and no agglutination on the test slide is a negative test. Agglutination on the control slide means an invalid test.

   Drying up of the solution must not be confused with agglutination.

Tube test

1. Place 2 drops of anti-D reagent in the tube labelled test.
2. Place 2 drops of normal saline or any other negative control reagent (no anti-D) in a tube labelled control.

3. Add 1-2 drops of 5% cell suspension in each tube.
4. Mix properly and incubate the tubes at 37°C for 10 minutes in an incubator or waterbath and then centrifuge at 1000 rpm for 1-2 minutes.
5. Disperse the cell button and observe for agglutination.
6. *Record the results:* Agglutination in the tube labeled test and smooth suspension in the control tube is a positive test while smooth suspension in both tubes is a negative test. Agglutination in the control tube is an invalid test.

Controls

It is always advisable to run parallel controls of known O Rh positive or O Rh negative cells along with all the Rh typing tests.

False positive

The agglutination may appear in the tube labelled test because of one of the following:

- Immunologically coated cells of patients.
- Contamination of antisera.
- Polyagglutination.
- The cells and antisera suspension left for a longer time.
  It is advisable to use two types of sera from two different manufacturers.

False negative

- Wrong reagent and not anti-D has been used.
- The reagent was not added at all.
- Weak expression of D antigen.

Test for D^u

The D^U is the weak expression of D antigen, which is detected only by indirect antiglobulin test (IAT). The anti-D sera used for this test must contain IgG, either monoclonal or polyclonal. The IgM sera are not recommended for this test.

Procedure

- Place 1 drop of anti-D serum in the tube labelled test.
- Place 1 drop of control reagent (without anti-D) in the tube labelled control.
- Add 5% cell suspension to both the tubes.
- Mix properly and incubate at 37°C for 30 minutes.

- Centrifuge at 1000 rpm for 1 minute.
- Disperse the cell button and examine for agglutination, if strong reaction is seen, the cells are Rh D positive.
- If no agglutination is seen in the test sample, wash the cells 3-4 times with saline and discard the supernatant.
- Add 2 drops of antiglobulin reagent (Coomb's serum). Mix properly and centrifuge at 1000 rpm for 1 minute.
- Disperse the cell button and examine for agglutination.
- *Record the results:* If the test sample shows agglutination and the control none, the test is POSITIVE for D^u
- If the test sample is negative, add IgG sensitised control cells, the test would show agglutination. It simply confirms the test result and the validity of the procedure.

Other blood group systems

chapter 4

Beside ABO and Rh there are other blood group systems, but of less clinical significance. Their testing is not carried out as a routine. The antibodies of this system have also been found causing haemolytic transfusion reaction (HTR) and haemolytic disease of newborn (HDN).

Some of the other blood group systems are mentioned below.

Lewis blood group system

There is a genetic interaction between Lewis and ABO genes. These antigens are manufactured by tissue cells and secreted into body fluids.

Lewis antigens

The Lewis phenotype is controlled by interaction of three sets of inherited genes, Le le, Se se and Hh.

The antigens are Le^a and Le^b.

Lewis antibodies

Lewis antibodies are cold reacting IgM antibodies which bind complement. They can cause hemolytic transfusion reaction. There are mainly two antibodies acting against two antigens.

Anti-Le^a

This antibody is found in secretor individuals who lack corresponding antigens, and are depicted as Le (a- b-).

Anti-Le^b

This antibody is also detected in (a- b-) individuals who are non- secretors.

Like anti-H the anti-Le^b reacts strongly with O and A_2 red cells. The A_1 and A_1B individuals are most likely to produce anti-Le^b.

The antibody does not cause HTR.

Lewis antigens become weaker in pregnancy. Since Lewis antibodies are IgM in nature, they are not capable of causing HDN.

Detection of Lewis antigens

- Take 2 test tubes and label them anti-Le^a and anti-Le^b.

- Place 1 drop of anti-Le^a and anti-Le^b in each tube.
- Add 1 drop of 5% cell suspension to be tested in each tube.
- Incubate at room temperature for 1 hour.
- Mix properly and examine for agglutination under microscope.

MNS blood group system

MN was the second blood group system discovered after ABO, by Landstiener and Levine in 1927. Walsh and Montgomery in 1947 described Ss system, which was found to be close to MN.

MNS antigens

The MNS antigens are well developed at the time of birth and can be detected on foetal cells. The four types of antigens of the system are M, N, S and S.

Antibodies of MNS system

Anti-M

It is a rare antibody and most often found in infants. It reacts best at room temperature. The antibody may be a mixture of IgM and IgG. The anti-M reacting at 37°C can cause HTR.

Anti-N

It is an IgM antibody that reacts at room temperature. Like anti-M this antibody too is not clinically significant and does not cause HTR and HDN.

Anti-S and Anti-s

These are warm reactive antibodies showing strong reaction in indirect Coombs' test (ICT). These are clinically significant antibodies leading to HTR and HDN.

P blood group system

Discovered by Landstiener and Levine in 1927.

Antigens

The main antigens of the system are P1 and P and rarely P_1k and P_2k.

Antibodies

Anti-P_1

It is a cold reactive IgM antibody, which is detected in the sera of P_2 individuals. This is a clinically insignificant antibody.

Anti-P

This antibody too reacts best at room temperature, inspite of being IgG in nature. It is found in the sera of Pk individuals. The anti-P is associated with habitual abortions. It may cause HTR.

Anti-PP_1Pk

The antibody is a complement binding antibody reacting at a wide range of temperature. It may be IgM or IgG in nature. This is found in rare p individuals. It may cause HTR.

Ii blood group system

The Ii system was discovered by Wiener, et al in 1956.

Antigens

The I antigen is present on the red cells of almost all individuals. Very rarely in the absence of I antigen, another antigen i may be present.

Antibodies

Anti-i

It is a cold reactive IgM antibody, which readily binds complement. It rarely causes HTR.

Anti-I

Anti-I is a cold reactive autoagglutinin. It has been detected in the sera of patients of infectious mononucleosis. The antibody is clinically insignificant.

Kell blood group system

The phenotypes of this system are common in whites but rare in Indians and Arabs.

Antigens

Usually the antigens are K and k but infrequently Kp^a and Kp^b may also be present.

Antibodies

The antibodies are anti-K, anti-k, anti-Kp^a and anti-Kp^b. These antibodies react mostly in ICT. They may cause HTR and mild degree of HDN.

Kidd blood group system

The blood group picks its name from a patient, Mrs Kidd, in whose serum the antibody was first discovered. The group was discovered by Allen, et al in 1951.

Antigens

The two types of antigens of the Kidd system are JK^a and JK^b.

Antibodies

Anti-JK^a and anti-JK^b are IgG antibodies, which bind complement and are detected by ICT only. The antibodies cause mild HDN and delayed HTR.

Duffy blood group system

Like Kidd this blood group system too owes its name to a patient, a haemophiliac, Mr Duffy, in whose serum Cutbush and Mollison detected the antibody in 1950.

Antigens

The antigens of the system are called Fy^a and Fy^b.

Antibodies

Anti-Fy^a and anti-Fy^b are warm reacting antibodies, detected by ICT. They are capable of causing HTR and HDN.

An association between Duffy blood group system and malaria has been observed. The Duffy individuals are found to be resistant to a West African malarial parasite; *Plasmodium knowlesi,* while the association with *P. vivax* is not well established.

Lutheran blood group system

The blood group system was discovered by Callender, et al in 1945.

Antigens

The antigens of this blood group system are Lu^a and Lu^b, which are rarely found in Indians.

Antibodies

Anti-Lu^a

This is a naturally occurring antibody reacting at room temperature. It does not cause HTR but may lead to mild HDN.

Anti-Lu^b

The antibody reacts in ICT and may cause HTR and mild HDN.

chapter 5

Antihuman globulin (Coombs') test

In 1946, Coombs and associates described the use of antihuman globulin to detect *in vivo* sensitisation of red cells in infants suffering from haemolytic disease of newborn (HDN). It was used for detection of weak incomplete antibodies present in the serum.

Principle of antiglobulin test

The incomplete antibodies are not capable of agglutinating the sensitised red cells on their own, since a gap remains between two sensitised cells.

The Fab portion of the incomplete antibody (IgG) binds with the sensitised red cells. When AHG (Coombs') serum is added the two Fab portions of the molecule (anti-IgG) attach to the Fc portions of the IgG antibodies, which have already attached to the red cells, and so, bridging the gap between sensitized cells causing agglutination **(Figure 5.1)**.

AHG (Coombs') reagents

The following types of AHG sera are available:

Polyspecific-1

The serum contains anti-IgG and anti-C3d. It may contain some more anticomplement or antiglobulin antibodies.

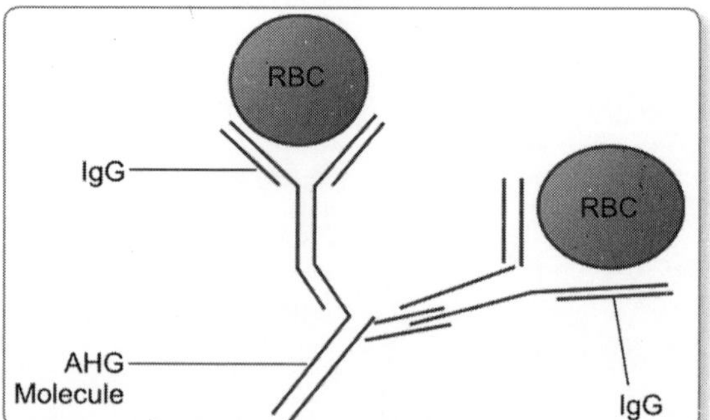

Figure 5.1 AHG molecule showing agglutination of RBC
(For colour version, see Plate 1)

Polyspecific-2

This reagent contains rabbit antihuman-IgG, monoclonal anti-C3b and C3d.

Monospecific anti-IgG

Contains only anti-IgG antibody with no complement activity.

Monospecific (Heavy chains)

The IgG antibodies present in this reagent are active only against gamma chains.

Anticomplement antibodies

It contains only anti-C3d and anti-C3b, but no anti-immunoglobulin.

Monoclonal antibodies

This reagent contains only anti- C3d (monoclonal) anti-C3b and- C3d (monoclonal). These antibodies react only against designated complement component.

The anti-IgM is not required in the AHG sera since it binds complements and anticomplement antibodies do that job.

Role of anticomplement antibodies

- To detect IgM antibodies which are complement binding.
- To detect complement binding antibodies of Duffy, Kell and Kidd systems.

AHG control cells

The AHG control cells are employed for confirmation of the test and to check the validity of the procedure in DAT and IAT.
Positive control is sensitised ORh + red cells.
Negative control is unsensitised ORh + red cells.

Preparation of positive control

To prepare the sensitised ORh+ cells in the laboratory, the following procedure is to be adopted:

- Take polyspecific anti-D serum and dilute it with normal saline, to the extent that, when treated with Rh positive cells, it just sensitizes the cells but does not lead to agglutination.

- Add 1 drop of 2-5% washed cell suspension of Rh+ cells to 2 drops of diluted anti-D serum.
- Incubate the mixture at 37°C for 30 minutes.
- If agglutination appears the anti-D serum is to be diluted further.
- Repeat the procedure with the rediluted anti-D serum.
- If no agglutination appears, wash the red cells three times in saline. Decant the supernatant completely every time. The prepared cells are sensitised cells.
- Make 5% cells suspension of the sensitised cells.
- Add 1 drop of AHG serum to 1 drop of 5% washed sensitised cells.
- Mix properly and centrifuge at 1000 rpm for 1 minute.
- Now the red cells should show agglutination, if no agglutination is seen that indicates the cells were not sensitised and the whole procedure is to be repeated with less diluted anti-D serum.

Gel card technique for Coombs' test

The microtubes of the ID-Card "LISS/Coombs" **(Figure 5.2)** contain polyspecific AHG, to be used for antibody screening, antibody identification, cross matching and the DAT. For IAT intensive washing procedures are eliminated.

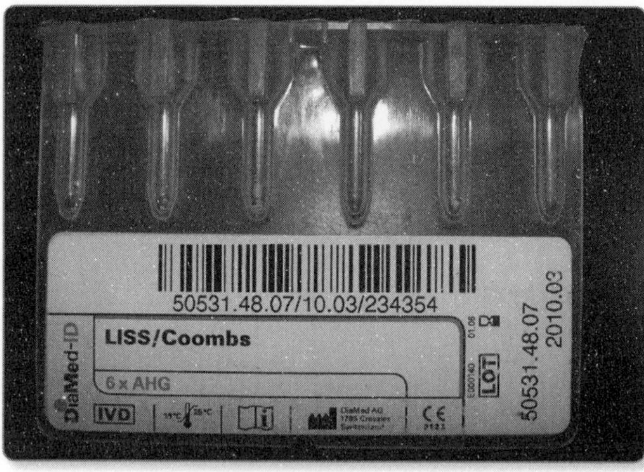

Figure 5.2: Gel card for DAT and IAT (Coombs' tests)
(For colour version, see Plate 2)

Additional reagents required

- ID-diluent: modified LISS for red cell suspension.
- ID-diacell, ID-diapanel: test cell reagents.

Materials required

- ID-dispenser
- ID-pipette
- ID-tips
- Suspension tubes
- ID-working table
- ID-incubator 37°C
- ID-card centrifuge.

Samples

The EDTA or citrate sample can be used.

a. Red cell suspension for DAT:
   Prepare a 0.8% red cell suspension in ID-diluent 2 as follows:
   - Allow the diluent to reach the room temperature before use.
   - Disperse 1.0 ml of ID-diluent 2 into a clean tube.
   - Add 10 μL of packed red cells, mix gently.

b. Plasma or serum for IAT.

Procedure

A. *Direct antiglobulin test (DAT):*
   1. Identify the appropriate microtubes of the ID-card "LISS/ Coombs" with the patient's or donor's name and number.
   2. Remove the aluminium foil from as many microtubes as required, holding the ID card in upright position.
   3. Pipette 50 μL of the red cell suspension to the appropriate microtube.
   4. Centrifuge the ID-card for 10 minutes in the ID-centrifuge.
   5. Read and record the results.

B. *Indirect antiglobulin test (IAT) and antibody screening:*

The ready to use ID DiaCell may be used.

1. Identify the appropriate microtubes of the ID-card LISS/Coombs with the patient's or donor's number and name.
2. Remove the aluminium foil from as many microtubes as required by holding the ID card in the upright position.
3. Pipette 50 μL of each test cell reagent to the appropriate microtube.

4. Pipette 50 µL of the sample's own red cell suspension to be used as autocontrol.
5. Add 25 µL of the patient's or donor's plasma or serum to each microtube.
6. Incubate the ID-card for 15 minutes at 37°C in the ID incubator.
7. Centrifuge the ID-card for 10 minutes in the ID centrifuge.
8. Read and record the results.

Clinical significance of Coombs' test

Direct antiglobulin test (DAT)

Principle

The DAT is applied to demonstrate the coating of IgG antibody or a complement component (C3d) on the surface of red cells, which is called sensitisation of red cells *in vivo.*

The DAT is diagnostic in the following conditions:
- Autoimmune hemolytic anaemia (AIHA).
- Hemolytic disease of the newborn (HDN).
- Investigation of haemolytic transfusion reaction (HTR).
- Investigation of drug-induced sensitisation.

Indirect antiglobulin test (IAT)

Principle

The IAT is applied for the detection of incomplete antibodies or complement binding antibodies found in the serum of the patient, after coating red cells *in vitro.*

The IAT is employed in the following conditions:
- Compatibility testing (Cross matching).
- Detection of unexpected alloantibodies in the serum.
- Detection of antigens of other blood group systems like Fy^a, Fy^b, JK^a, JK^b and Le^a, etc.

Procedure of DAT/DCT

The blood sample for DAT should be collected in EDTA.
- Place 1-2 drops of washed 5% cell suspension to be tested in a test tube.
- Add 1-2 drops of polyspecific AHG serum.

- Mix and centrifuge at 1000 rpm for 1 minute.
- Disperse the cell button.
- Examine for agglutination. Confirm all negative tests under microscope
- Record the result.
- If the test result is non-reactive, leave it for 5 minutes at RT and read again.
- If the test appears negative, add 1 drop of positive control (sensitised ORh+ cells). Mix and centrifuge at 1000 rpm for 1 minute.

Agglutination should appear now, if still no agglutination is seen, the test is invalid and the whole procedure should be repeated.

Interpretation

If the agglutination appears at step 5 or 7, the DAT is positive.

In case the number of IgG molecules is less than 500 the chances are that, they will not be picked up by polyspecific AHG sera. In this case even though the cells are coated by antibodies, the DAT may appear negative.

Procedure of IAT/ICT

The sample for IAT must be fresh for detection of complement binding antibodies. IAT is performed on the sera of patient or donor.

- Place 2 drops of the test serum in a test tube.
- Add 1 drop of 5% washed cell suspension of the donor/patient.
- Mix gently and incubate at 37°C for 30 minutes.
- Centrifuge the mixture at 1000 rpm for 1 minute.
- Observe for agglutination. If no agglutination is seen at this stage, proceed further.
- Wash the cells at least 3 times and decant the supernatant completely.
- Add 1 drop of polyspecific AHG serum.
- Centrifuge at 1000 rpm for 1 minute.
- Disperse the cell button and examine for agglutination.
- If the result is still non-reactive, leave the mixture at RT for 5 minutes.
- Record the results. Examine all negative tests under microscope.

Add 1 drop of positive control (sensitised Rh+ O cells) to the non-reactive sample. Mix and centrifuge at 1000 rpm for 1 minute. The agglutination must appear at this stage, otherwise the procedure is invalid and must be repeated.

Interpretation

If agglutination is seen at step 5, it shows presence of saline reacting antibodies. If agglutination appears at step 11, the IAT is positive.

Factors affecting AHG test

Ratio of serum to cell

By increasing the ratio of serum to cell the degree of antibody coating on cells can be increased. Ideal ratio is 1 drop of cells to 2 drops of serum.

Temperature

The antigen antibody association decreases at lower temperature. The ideal temperature for reaction is 37°C.

Incubation time

The optimum incubation time for saline or enzyme medium is 30 minutes. This period can be raised in cases of weak reacting antibodies.

Reaction medium

The sensitivity of IAT is increased by adding 22% bovine albumin or enzyme (papain) or low ionic strength solution (LISS).

Albumin IAT technique

The intensity of reaction of antigen antibody is increased and incubation time is reduced with addition of 22% bovine albumin in IAT.

Procedure

It is performed either by one stage or two stage method.

One stage method

In one stage method, 2 drops of 22% bovine albumin is added along with cell suspension at step 2, which reduces the incubation time to 20 minutes. The rest of the procedure is same as in IAT.

Two stage method

Add 2 drops of 22% albumin after incubation at step 3 of IAT and then incubate again for 15-20 minutes. Proceed further as in IAT from step 4 onwards.

Enzyme IAT technique

The enzymes increase the clustering of antigenic sites as well as reduce the negative charge on the red cell surface.

Procedure

Add 1 drop of enzyme papain in step 2 of IAT along with the cell suspension. Proceed further from step 3 as of saline IAT.

Sources of error

False positive

The result of AHG test may appear false positive in the following conditions:

- Cells may be autoagglutinable.
- Cells positive for DAT used for IAT.
- Contamination of cells or saline.
- Overcentrifugation.
- Polyagglutination.
- Dirty glassware.

False negative

The result of AHG test may appear false negative in the following conditions:

- Inadequate washing of cells.
- AHG reagent non-reactive.
- AHG reagent not added.
- Serum not added in IAT.
- Inadequate incubation.
- Cell suspension either too weak or too heavy.
- Under centrifugation.

Detection and identification of antibodies

chapter 6

Antibody detection and identification is one of the most challenging aspects of immunohaematology. The proficiency of the technique acts as "icing on the cake". In routine practice, the blood banking consists of ABO and Rh testing, antibody screening and cross matching procedures. The unexpected antibodies may pose a problem for the blood bank staff at one of the following phases of compatibility test:

- Immediate spin at RT.
- Albumin or enzyme phase at 37°C.
- Indirect antiglobulin test.

The screening of the antibodies is carried out in the recipients, donors or antenatal patients. Early detection of the antibody in the serum of the mother may help the paediatrician in taking a decision in favour of intrauterine or exchange transfusion in the neonate.

If unexpected antibodies are detected during compatibility testing, one of the two courses of action may be considered, depending on the facilities available in the blood bank.

If the blood bank is well equipped, identify the antibody with the help of panel of screening cells. Select a blood unit which lacks the corresponding antigen.

If the screening cells are not available, the cross matching is to be carried out with several donor units until a compatible blood is found.

Screening cells

The screening cells are of two types:

Primary panel

The primary panel is consisting of two or three types of 3% group O cells in homozygous form, known as OR_1R_1, OR_2R_2 and OR_3R_3 which carry the main antigens of Rh, Duffy, Kell, Kidd, MNSs, P and Lewis **(Figures 6.1** and **6.2)**. These cells are used for preliminary screening of antibodies.

Secondary panel

The secondary panel of cells is consisting of 3% suspension of 11 group O cells, which are collected from different donors. These cells carry

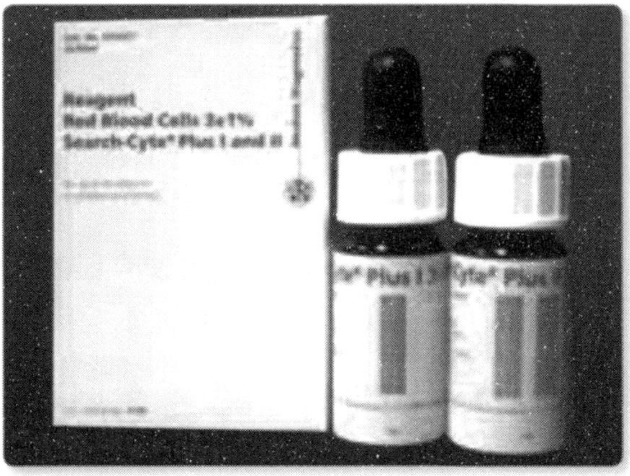

Figure 6.1 Two donor's primary panel of cells
(For colour version, see Plate 2)

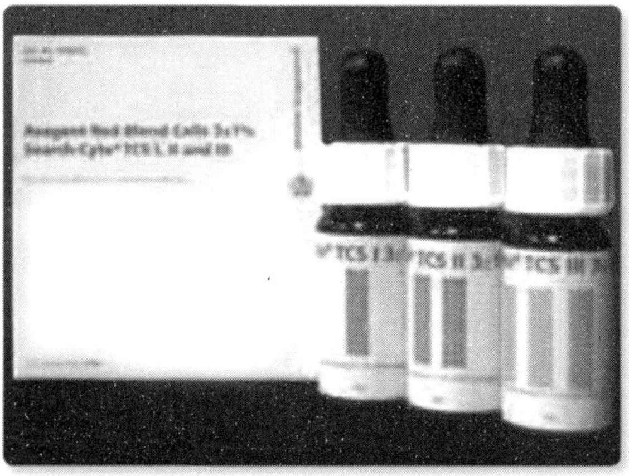

Figure 6.2 Three donor's primary panel of cells
(For colour version, see Plate 3)

maximum number of antigens namely, D, C, E, c, e, K, k, Fy^a, Fy^b, M, N, S, s, JK^a, JK^b, P, Le^a, Le^b, Lu^a and Lu^b **(Figure 6.3)**. The panel of screening cells is commercially available, but it can also be prepared in the laboratory. These cells are carefully selected to allow the easy identification of both individual antibodies and combination of antibodies.

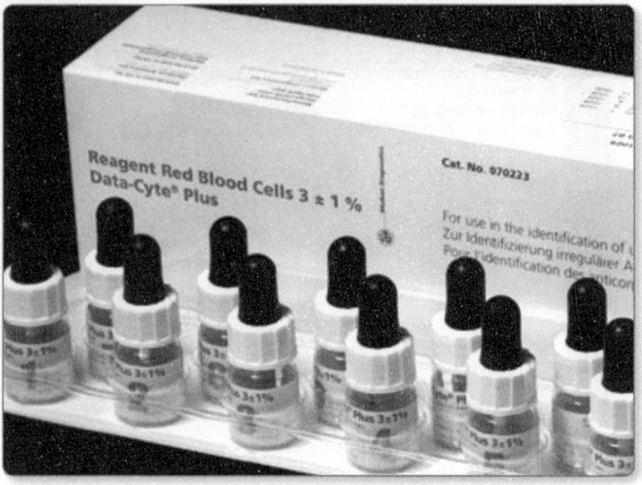

Figure 6.3 Secondary panel of antibodies screening cells
(For colour version, see Plate 3)

Panel of monospecific antibodies reacting against antigens of Rh and all other group antigens are also commercially available.

Detection of antibodies

The initial detection of antibodies is done by primary panel of screening cells, applying them to all the three phases of testing, saline, enzyme and IAT. A parallel run of autocontrol with the cells and serum of the same individual is advisable. Agglutination or haemolysis is recorded as positive test. The results are scored and interpreted accordingly by short-listing the antibodies (Table 6.1).

Identification of alloantibodies

When the antibodies have been detected in the preliminary testing by primary panel, the next course of action is to identify the specific antibody with the help of secondary panel of cells **(Figure 6.4)**.

Before proceeding with identification of antibodies, proper medical history including H/O transfusion, pregnancy and drug intake should be reviewed.

All the preliminary tests of ABO grouping and subgrouping, Rh typing and DAT must also be repeated.

Table 6.1: Some of the results of antibody detection tests

Cell	IS	37°C	AGT
SC I	neg	neg	neg
SC II	neg	neg	2+
Auto	neg	neg	neg
1. *Single alloantibody*			
2. *Probably IgG antibody*			
Cell	**IS**	**37°C**	**AGT**
SC I	neg	1+	3+
SC II	neg	neg	1+
Auto	neg	neg	neg
1. *Multiple antibodies*			
2. *Single antibody*			
3. *IgG antibody*			
Cell	**IS**	**37°C**	**AGT**
SC I	1+	neg	neg
SC II	2+	neg	neg
Auto	neg	neg	neg
1. *Single or multiple antibody*			
2. *IgM antibody*			
Cell	**IS**	**37°C**	**AGT**
SC I	neg	neg	3+
SC II	neg	neg	3+
Auto	neg	neg	3+
1. *Warm antibody*			
2. *Probably IgG antibody*			
3. *Transfusion reaction*			

SC = screening cells; IS = immediate spin; AGT = Antiglobulin test

The identification of antibodies is based on the results of detection tests. The investigator should consider the following questions:

- In what phase did the reactions occur?
- Is the autocontrol positive or negative ?
- Is haemolysis there?
- Whether agglutination is true or it is only rouleaux phenomenon.

	Rh								MNS				Lutheran		P1		Lewis		Kell		Duffy		Kidd		Liss		Check
Cell	D	C	E	c	e	f	V	C^w	M	N	S	s	Lu^a	Lu^b	P_1	P_1	Le^a	Le^b	K	k	Fy^a	Fy^b	Jk^a	Jk^b	ALC	AHC	Cells
1. r'r-2	0	0	0	+	+	+	0	0	+	+	0	+	0	+	0	0	0	+	0	+	+	0	+	+	θ	2+	
2. $R1^wR1$-1	+	+	0	0	+	0	0	+	+	+	+	0	+	+	+	+	0	+	0	+	0	+	+	0	θ	2+	
3. R1R1-6	+	+	0	0	+	0	0	0	0	+	0	+	0	+	+	+	+	0	+	+	0	+	+	0	θ	2+	
4. R2R2-8	+	0	+	+	0	0	0	0	+	+	+	+	0	+	+	+	0	+	+	0	0	+	0	+	θ	θ	✓
5. R"4-3	0	0	+	+	+	+	0	0	+	+	+	0	0	+	+	+	+	0	0	0	0	+	0	+	θ	θ	✓
6. rr-32	0	0	0	+	+	+	+	+	+	0	+	0	0	+	+	+	0	0	0	0	0	+	+	0	θ	θ	✓
7. rr-10	0	0	0	+	+	+	0	0	+	+	+	+	0	+	0	0	0	+	+	+	0	+	+	+	θ	θ	✓
8. rr-12	0	0	0	+	+	+	0	0	0	+	0	+	0	+	+	+	0	+	0	+	+	0	0	+	θ	θ	✓
9. R_0-4	+	0	0	+	+	+	0	0	+	0	0	+	0	+	0	0	+	0	0	+	0	0	0	+	θ	θ	✓
Cord cell																	0	0									
Patient																									θ	θ	✓

Direct antihuman globulin test

Poly	negative
IgG	
C3	

Figure 6.4 Antigram showing presence of anti-C antibody

The next step is application of secondary panel of cells. The antigram provided with the panel would reveal what antigens are present on which number of cells. Manufacturer's instructions must be followed. It is advisable to have parallel run of patient's own cells as autocontrol and two group O Rh positive and negative cord cells along with the panel cells. The cord cells have i antigen while I is missing.

Procedure

The patient's serum is to be tested against panel cells, own cells and cord cells in all the three following phases:

- Immediate spin or saline phase (at RT).
- Enzyme phase (37°C).
- Indirect antiglobulin test (IAT).

Saline phase

1. Take 14 test tubes, 11 for panel of cells (depending on number of cells), 1 for autocontrol and 2 for cord cells.
2. Place 2 drops of patient's serum in each tube.
3. Add 1 drop of panel cell 1 in tube 1 and continue with corres-ponding cells to the labelled tubes up to tube 11. Add 1 drop of patient's own cell suspension in tube 12 and 1 drop each of cord cell suspension in tube 13 and 14.
4. Mix gently and incubate at RT for 1 hour.
5. Shake the tubes and dislodge the button.
6. Haemolysis at this stage must be considered positive test.
7. Examine all negative results microscopically.
8. Score and record the result on the antigram chart provided with the panel.

Enzyme phase

1. Add 1 drop of enzyme papain in each tube just after the step 2 of saline test.
2. Incubate at 37°C for 1 hour.
3. The rest of the steps are same as of saline test.

IAT

The test would detect warm IgG and complement binding antibodies.

Follow the exact procedure of IAT as described earlier on all the 14 tubes.

Score and record the results of enzyme and IAT on the antigram chart.

Evaluation of panel results

Start from negative tests. Strike out all the antigens which are present on the cells but show no agglutination or haemolysis in all the three phases.

When you have ruled out the antigenic determinate present on all the panel cells, note down the remaining antigens. They may be one or more than one.

Record the result

The remaining antigen would confirm the corresponding antibody reacting against it. For example, if the chart shows that C or E is the only remaining antigen reacting, so the corresponding antibody present in the patient's serum is either anti-C or anti-E.

Cross-matching (compatibility testing)

chapter 7

The basic principle of the modern day transfusion therapy is, that it should provide maximum benefit with none or minimum risk to the patient. As the knowledge of the new blood group systems and sophisticated methods for antibody detection increased, so did the search for more sensitive compatibility methods.

The compatibility testing includes, ABO and Rh typing on the donor and recipient blood samples, screening of donor's and patient's sera for unexpected alloantibody, and finally a cross-match.

Cross-matching

The cross-matching is of two types: major cross-match and minor cross-match.

Major cross-match

When the donor's red cells and the patient's serum is mixed and tested, it is called major cross-match: Donor's cells + Patient's serum.

Minor cross-match

Donor's serum + Patient's cells.

Sample collection for cross-matching

The blood sample from the patient must be collected in both, EDTA and plain tubes, in order to perform forward and reverse grouping.

If detection of alloantibodies in the patient's serum is to be carried out, at least 5 ml blood sample in a plain vial is required.

The donor sample is collected from the pilot tube or one of the segments of the tube attached to the bag. The number given on the segment should always be recorded for proper identification.

Procedure of cross-matching for whole blood transfusion

Saline technique

This technique is designed to detect IgM antibodies of ABO system.

- Label two test tubes, one A for major and one B for minor cross-match.
- Place 2 drops of patient's serum in the tube labelled A and 2 drops of donor's serum in the tube labelled B.
- Add 1 drop of 2-5% (tomato coloured) cell suspension of the donor in tube A and 1 drop of patient's cells in tube B.
- Mix and incubate at RT for 10 minutes.
- Centrifuge at 1000 rpm for 1-2 minutes.
- Place 1 drop from each tube A and B on two separate glass slides and examine under microscope.
- Put a drop of saline on each slide to disperse the rouleaux.
- Record the results.

Interpretation

Haemolysis or even weak agglutination (2-3 cells sticking together) is considered incompatible **(Figure 7.1)**.

Albumin and AHG technique

The addition of 22% albumin acts as an enhancing medium. When it is incorporated along with IAT in cross-matching, it helps in detection of weak reacting antibodies and also IgG antibodies reacting at 37°C.

Single tube cross-match

In most of the blood banks where whole blood is rarely used and only the major cross-matching is performed, the technique of single tube cross-match is employed.

Procedure

Saline phase

- Place 2 drops of patient's serum in a test tube.
- Add 1 drop of 2-5% washed cell suspension of the donor.
- Mix and incubate at RT for 10 minutes.
- Centrifuge at 1000 rpm for 1 minute.
- Resuspend the cell button. Agglutination at this stage indicates presence of IgM antibodies.

Albumin phase

- Add 1-2 drops of 22% bovine albumin to the serum cell mixture.
- Incubate at 37°C for 30 minutes.
- Centrifuge at 1000 rpm for 1 minute.
- Haemolysis or agglutination at this stage indicates presence of weak reacting (IgG) antibodies.
- Wash the cells three times with normal saline and discard the supernatant completely every time.

AHG/ IAT phase

- Add 2 drops of AHG serum.
- Centrifuge at 1000 rpm for 1 minute.
- Dislodge the button gently and examine for agglutination.
- Haemolysis or agglutination at this stage indicates presence of IgG antibodies.

Interpretation

A blood donor unit is labelled fully compatible with the patient's blood when no agglutination is observed in none of the three phases of the compatibility testing **(Figure 7.1)**.

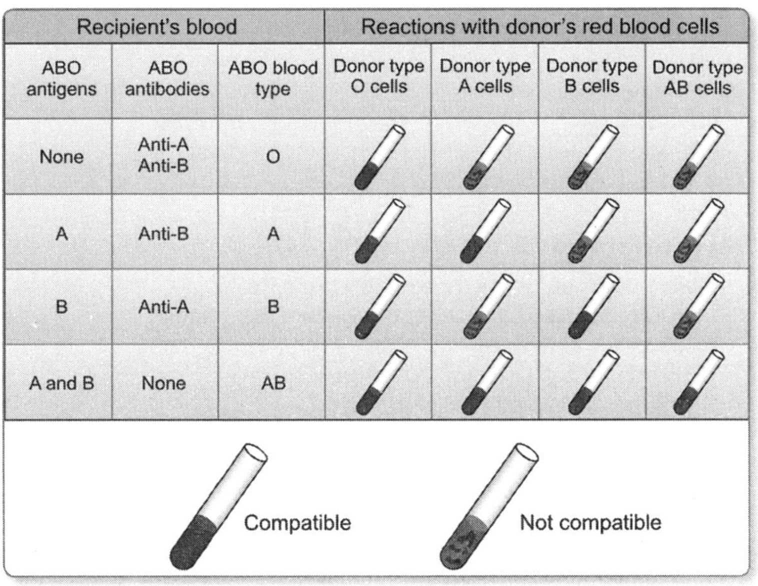

Figure 7.1 Diagrammatic presentation of ABO compatibility
(For colour version, see Plate 4)

Cross-matching in emergencies

The procedure is carried out in accidental cases where, there is no time for proper cross-matching.

Procedure

- Test recipient's sample for ABO and Rh grouping.
- Arrange group specific donor unit.
- Mix 1 drop of 5% cell suspension of donor with 2 drops of patient's serum.
- Centrifuge for 2-5 minutes.
- If O Rh negative blood is being used, switch over to group specific blood after O group transfusion of two units of whole blood or six units of RBC concentrate.
- Blood issued before complete cross-matching procedure must be labelled "uncross-matched blood" and the cross-matching procedure should be completed afterwards as soon as possible.

Low ionic strength salt (LISS)

The LISS reduces the electrostatic barrier surrounding red cells and increases the rate of antibody uptake to four folds compared to normal saline. It results in increase in the antibody titre and reduced incubation period.

LISS solution contains:

- 0.17 M saline 180 ml
- 0.15 M phosphate buffer, pH 6.7 20 ml
- 0.3 M sodium glycinate, pH 6.7 800 ml

Procedure (rapid 15 minutes test)

- Place 2 drops of patient's serum in a test tube.
- Add 2 drops of 5% LISS suspended cells of the donor.
- Incubate for 15 minutes at 37°C.
- Centrifuge at 1000 rpm for 1-2 minutes.
- Check for haemolysis or agglutination.
- Wash the cells 3 times in normal saline and discard the supernatant completely.
- Add 1-2 drops of AHG serum.
- Centrifuge and look for agglutination.
- Add IgG coated (positive control) cells to negative AHG test.
- Agglutination should appear at this stage.

Interpretation

If there is no agglutination at step 5 or 8, the donor unit is labelled compatible with patient's blood.

Procedure for issuing blood unit

The technician while issuing the blood must ensure that the label on the unit contains the following information:

- Donor's registration number.
- Donor's blood group (ABO and Rh).
- Date of collection.
- Date of expiry.
- Stamp designating HBsAg, anti-HCV, HIV_1 and HIV_2, VDRL/RPR/TPHA and Malaria (anti-HBc and also $HTLV_1$, where applicable) negative.
- Name of the person who cross-matched blood.
- Name of the patient/ recipient.
- Patient's blood group.
- Date and time of issue.

Recheck the date of expiry, screening status, donor's and patient's identification and the blood unit for abnormal colour or signs of haemolysis.

Transfusion reactions and complications

chapter 8

The blood is a complex product and its transfusion to a complex organism; the patient, occasionally causes adverse effects which are commonly known as transfusion reactions. Some of the transfusion reactions are unavoidable while some are preventable.

Types of transfusion reactions

The transfusion reactions are classified in two ways:
Classification based on the type of reaction:

A. Haemolytic transfusion reactions
B. Nonhaemolytic transfusion reactions

Alternatively, the transfusion reactions are classified based on time taken for the reactions to appear.

a. Immediate adverse effects
b. Delayed adverse effects.

Haemolytic transfusion reactions (HTR)

The HTR takes place due to incompatibility of red cells leading to immunological destruction of cells called haemolysis. The haemolysis may be either:

- Intravascular haemolysis; due to ABO incompatibility, or
- Extravascular haemolysis; due to incompatibility of Rh or occasionally K, k S or Fy systems.

The haemolytic transfusion reactions are clinically most signi-ficant. They may be fatal if not detected early and managed properly. Almost all haemolytic transfusion reactions can be prevented.

The causes of HTR are as follows:

- *Clerical errors*
  - Misidentification of the recipient: At the time of collection of blood sample for cross-matching or at the time of transfusion.
  - Incorrect or inadequate labelling of blood samples of the recipient, donor unit or pilot tube.
- *Technical errors*
  - Error in blood grouping of the recipient or donor sample

- Error in cross-matching procedure and incompatibility not detected.
- Inadequate cross-matching where weak or IgG antibodies go undetected.
- Transfusion of multiple units of O group whole blood to A or B individual leading to haemolysis of red cells of the recipient by the antibodies of the donor.

Events in haemolytic transfusion reaction

The signs and symptoms of HTR are manifested in four phases, if not managed promptly.

The four phases are as follows:

1. *Shock phase*
   This is the earliest phase. The signs and symptoms are fever with chill, perspiration, pain in the chest and back, haemorrhage and shock.
2. *Postshock phase*
   The patient shows signs of:
   - Haemoglobinaemia
   - Haemoglobinuria
   - Hyperbilirubinaemia, and
   - If not managed, the patient lands up in Disseminated Intra-vascular Coagulation (DIC).
3. *Anuric phase*
   From the postshock phase the patient proceeds to anuric phase and shows signs of renal failure like anuria and uraemia.
4. *Recovery phase*
   After approximately 8 to 12 days, the renal functions start returning to normal. The blood urea, creatinine and potassium levels come down.

Role of transfusionist in HTR

If the haemolytic transfusion reaction is suspected, the transfusionist must take the following steps:

- Stop the transfusion immediately.
- Keep the intravenous (IV) line patent with IV fluids.
- Recheck the records of the patient, the labels on the blood unit to establish the identity of the patient and the donor unit.
- Collect patient's post-transfusion blood and urine samples and send them to blood bank.
- Return the blood bag with the remaining blood to the blood bank.

Investigation of a case of transfusion reaction

If a transfusion reaction is reported, the first job of the blood bank staff is to determine the type of the reaction; whether it is haemolytic or non-haemolytic. Since HTR is a serious condition and occurs mostly due to clerical or technical error, hence the responsibility is to be fixed.

The investigation should proceed in the following steps:

- Recheck all the documents, the identity of the patient, donor unit, pilot tube and the cross-matching record to ensure there was no clerical error.
- Examine the patient's pretransfusion and post-transfusion sample for any change of colour of plasma or serum. If the plasma or serum in the post transfusion sample appears red, it is an indication of haemolysis.
- Repeat the ABO and Rh blood grouping on the patient's pre- and post-transfusion samples, pilot tube or the remaining segment on the blood bag.
- Cross-match again the patient's pre- and post-transfusion blood samples with the blood in the pilot segment of tube of the bag, and with the remaining blood in the bag.
- Perform direct antiglobulin test (DAT) on the patient's red cells from the post-transfusion sample.

Interpretation of the results

- If no discrepancy is found in the pretransfusion and post-transfusion grouping and cross-matching results, and the DAT is negative, it indicates that no HTR has taken place.
- If the patient's condition suggests HTR and the results of investigations show incompatibility and the DAT is positive, the following confirmatory tests should be carried out.
  - *Test for haemoglobinaemia:* Test of free haemoglobin in the patient's post transfusion plasma sample.
  - *Test for hyperbilirubinaemia:* Nonconjugated bilirubin is tested in the serum of the post transfusion sample.
  - *Test for haemoglobinuria:* The post-transfusion urine sample is tested for presence of haemoglobin.
  - If the HTR is established, the next step is to identify the antibody responsible for the reaction.
  - Antibody screening test is done in patient's pre- and post- transfusion samples by the primary panel of screening cells.
  - If an unexpected antibody is detected, the identification of the antibody is done by the secondary panel of cells, in saline, enzyme and IAT phases.

- Finally the donor's blood cells lacking the corresponding antigen are crossmatched with the patient's serum.

Nonimmunological causes of haemolysis

The haemolysis of the transfused red cells may occur due to the following non-immunological causes:

- Physical destruction of blood cells due to freezing or overheating.
- Mixing of nonisotonic solutions with red cells.

Non-haemolytic transfusion reactions

The various types of non-haemolytic transfusion reactions and the factors responsible for them are given below:

Leucocyte incompatibility

Febrile reactions

These reactions occur during or within one hour of transfusion resulting in rise of body temperature with chills. The granulocyte antibodies, HLA or lymphocyte reactive antibodies may bear the major etiologic responsibility, possibly by release of interleukin-1.

Noncardiac pulmonary reactions

The reaction occurs due to leukocyte aggregates trapped in the pulmonary microcirculation.

Mild febrile reactions can be managed by antipyretics.

The choice of component for transfusion in these circumstances is leucocyte poor blood.

Reactions due to plasma proteins

The antibodies to the plasma proteins cause urticaria in patients.

Platelet incompatibility

Febrile reactions

The fever and chill may also be because of antibodies to the platelets in a patient who has received many units of platelets from different donors.

Post-transfusion purpura

Some of the patients develop a platelet specific antibody; antihuman platelet antibody (anti-HPA) which destroys platelets leading to thrombocytopenia. It manifests as pupuric rashes.

Anaphylactic reactions

The anaphylactic reactions presenting as flushing of face, vomiting, respiratory distress and shock may occur due to anti-IgA in IgA deficient patients.

Allergic reactions

If the patient already has reagins, they would react with the transfused allergens resulting in wheal formation, laryngeal edema or bronchial spasm.

Transfusion-related acute lung injury (TRALI)

The acute lung injury occurring within six hours following a transfusion is known as TRALI. Its a serious complication of transfusion characterized by noncardiogenic pulmonary oedema. TRALI is the cause of most transfusion related fatalities.

TRALI is an immune mediated disorder. Antibodies directed toward HLA are the most probable cause of TRALI. Multiparous women are more prone to suffer from TRALI.

Transfusion reactions based on time factor

Immediate effects

The adverse effects or reactions, which occur during transfusion or within few hours of transfusion, are known as immediate adverse effects of transfusion.

Some immediate effects are:

- Haemolysis: Either due to red cell incompatibility or physical destruction of RBC.
- Febrile nonhaemolytic reactions due to leukocyte incompatibility.
- Urticaria.
- Anaphylaxis.
- Fever with shock due to bacterial contamination of blood.
- Volume overload leading to congestive heart failure.

Delayed effects

- The adverse effects of transfusion, which take days to months to manifest, are known as delayed effects. This includes diseases transmitted through transfusion.

Some of the delayed effects are mentioned below:

- Haemolysis due to secondary response of antibodies to red cells.
- Primary alloimmunisation because of exposure to donor antigens.
- Post-transfusion purpura.
- Graft vs host disease (GvHD).
- Iron overload, because of multiple transfusions; commonly seen in thalassaemics.
- Malaria.
- Hepatitis B and C, and rarely A.
- Syphilis.
- AIDS.
- Mononucleosis due to Cytomegalovirus (CMV) or Epstein Bar Virus (EBV).

Screening for diseases transmitted through blood

chapter 9

Blood transfusion is given as a life-saving measure, but the chances of transmission of microorganisms remains a potential danger. The diseases and viruses transmitted as a result of transfusion of blood are known as transfusion transmitted diseases (TTD) and transfusion transmitted viruses (TTV). Rigid criteria for the selection of donor and the availability of sophisticated screening procedures have considerably reduced the possibility of TTD, but the risk has been only minimized not ruled out. The best policy still remains to avoid transfusion, unless its benefits outdo the risks.

The screening of donor's blood is carried out for the following TTDs:

- Hepatitis B
- Hepatitis C
- Syphilis
- AIDS
- Malaria.

Some of the infrequently transmitted diseases are as follows:
Hepatitis G, Brucellosis, Toxoplasmosis and other viral infections—Human T Lymphotropic Virus 1 (HTLV1), Cytomegalovirus (CMV) and Epstein bar virus (EBV).

Tests for hepatitis B

Transmission of hepatitis B by blood is a common and serious complication. Transmission of hepatitis A is very rare because of its short incubation period and almost absence of carrier state. The test for hepatitis A is not part of a routine pretransfusion testing.

The first marker, which appears in cases of hepatitis B, is hepatitis B surface antigen (HBsAg).This marker is also detectable in chronic carriers. Antihepatitis B core antibody (Anti-HBc) is also detected in acute phase as well as during window period.

The following tests are available in order of sensitivity for detection of HBsAg:

- Immunodiffusion
- Enzyme-linked Immunosorbent Assay (ELISA) and Radio- immuno Assay (RIA)

- Counter electrophoresis
- Latex agglutination
- Complement fixation tests
- Passive haemagglutination inhibition.

The test procedure must be performed according to manufacturer's instructions.

Rapid tests

The rapid tests are available for HBsAg, anti-HCV, HIV 1 and 2 and for syphilis. The authors have reported a sensitivity and specificity of more than 99% for these kits. These kits are recommended only in cases of emergencies and special circumstances, otherwise testing for all the transfusion transmitted diseases (TTD) must be performed by ELISA technique only.

Reagent

Rapid HBsAg test is a ready to use suspension of latex particles. The latex particles are coated with IgG monoclonal anti-HBs antibodies.

Procedure

All the samples and the reagents are to be brought at room temperature before testing.

- Place one drop of the test sample on the glass slide by the pipette provided.
- Prepare a 1:40 dilution of the samples in an isotonic saline.
- Pipette one drop of the diluted sample on the next reaction circle of the glass slide.
- Place one drop of the positive and negative controls onto the remaining reaction circles of the slide.
- After shaking the vial place one drop of the latex reagent to each sample including controls.
- Mix thoroughly using different sticks.
- Rock the slides gently back and forth.
- Observe for agglutination after 5 minutes.

Interpretation	*Result*
No agglutination with diluted and neat samples	Negative (HBsAg absent)
Agglutination with either neat or diluted sample, or with both samples	Positive (HBsAg present)

Test for anti-HCV antibody

Rapid kits are available in the market but the test by ELISA are recommended and now performed in every blood bank.

Screening tests for HIV1 and HIV2

One of the following screening tests for HIV may be performed in the blood bank.

- Dot blot assays
- Particle agglutination
- HIV spot and coombs' test.

ELISA

The test is sensitive, specific and cost effective. National AIDS Control Organization (NACO) recommends that all the tests for HIV in the blood bank should be performed by ELISA.

Simple test based on ELISA:

For all the above procedures different kits are available in the market.

If the donor tests positive, he is deferred from donating blood, and referred to Voluntary counseling and testing centre (VCTC) for counseling, and, if required he undergoes the confirmatory western blot test.

Test for syphilis

One of the following tests is performed for the screening of *Trepanoma pallidum* of syphilis on the donor's blood:

- Venereal Disease Research Laboratory (VDRL)
- Rapid plasma reagin (RPR)
- *Trepanoma pallidum* haemagglutination assay (TPHA).

Malaria

Various procedures are available for testing of malarial parasite in the blood bank.

The tests for HTLV1, anti-HBc, CMV, etc. depend on the regulations of the particular country. The ELISA kits are available for these tests.

Manufacturer's instructions provided with the kits must be followed for the procedures of the tests.

Blood donor and collection of blood

chapter 10

The blood donor

All "fresh" blood components and manufactured blood products originate from the blood donor. Hence, the safety of blood transfusion begins with careful selection of donors.

To protect both, the donor and the recipient, from any ill effects, donors must be in good health.

Types of Donors

- *Voluntary blood donor:* The person who donates blood not for any particular patient and seeks nothing in return is called a voluntary donor. The incidence of transfusion-transmitted diseases is much less in blood drawn from voluntary donors. They are the best type of donors and act as the lifeline of any blood transfusion service.
- *Replacement blood donor:* The donor who donates blood as a replacement for some of his relative or friend is a replacement donor. The majority of the blood supply in the blood banks of developing countries comes from replacement donors.
- *Professional blood donor:* The blood donors who seek benefit for their donation of blood in cash or kind are professional donors. Such donors are likely to hide correct information about their health status and may carry some infection. They are discouraged in most of the countries. In India, collection of blood from professional donors is prohibited by the judgment of the Supreme Court.

Only voluntary donors, with or without replacement should be accepted.

Registration of donor

This is mandatory for the blood banks to keep complete record of the blood donor, so the donor could be traced, in case he belongs to a rare blood group or for medicolegal purposes. The following record of the donor is to be maintained:

- Date of donation
- Name of donor
- Father's or husband's name
- Age
- Sex

- Occupation
- Complete workplace and residential addresses with phone numbers
- Date of last donation
- Previous donor reactions, if any
- Blood group
- If he has previously donated; results of the screening tests of TTD or if carrier of any alloantibody.
- Registration number (The blood bank allots a number to each registered donor).

Consent of donor

The written consent of the donor should be taken prior to the donation on the questionnaire itself. The format of the consent should be as follows:

"I have been explained the benefits of the transfusion and the minimum risks of donor reactions and I willingly and voluntarily agree to donate a unit of blood."

Signature or thumb impression of the donor................Date and time.

Selection of donor

Complete and extensive medical examination cannot be performed on every volunteer. Much reliance is therefore placed on answers to questions about his general health, medical history, and drugs being taken. Simple physical examination of the donor, and selected laboratory tests on his blood sample, are also carried out to ensure the safety of the donation for the recipient. Several other factors concern the health and wellbeing of the donor.

Medical history

A printed questionnaire pertaining to the medical history based on the following guidelines should be available in every blood bank. The literate donors should be encouraged to fill up the questionnaire themselves. The form contains space for the donor's consent. Based on his medical history, the medical officer decides whether the donor is accepted or deferred. The document should be treated confidential.

- The donor should be in sound mental state.
- The donor should not be fasting. It has been observed that hypoglycemia precipitates adverse donor reactions.
- History of past illness
- The donor is deferred if he gives a positive history of any of the following illness:

History of allergic disorders, epilepsy, renal, cardiovascular, malignant diseases, bleeding tendency, fainting, tuberculosis, and diabetes mellitus, or any other major illness.

Medication

Drugs present in the donor's bloodstream may adversely affect a recipient. The h/o any drug intake could indicate underlying illness, which in itself is a reason to defer the donor. If the donor is on antibiotics, antimalarials or antihypertensives, he is not accepted. If the donor has consumed salicylates (Aspirin) in the last 48 hours and his blood is going to be used for preparation of platelet concentrate, then he should be deferred.

Pregnancy

Pregnancy and at least six months during lactation makes a case for deferral.

Surgery

The donor is not accepted, six months after having gone through major surgery and three months after minor surgical procedures.

The donor who has himself received blood or blood component during the last six months is not accepted.

Immunisation

Hepatitis B vaccination

In case of prophylactic vaccination for hepatitis B the donor is accepted, but vaccination post-exposure is the cause for deferral for six months. If donor has received hepatitis B immunoglobulin then he is deferred for one year.

A symptom free donor is accepted, if he has been vaccinated with the following killed vaccines or toxoids:

- Vaccinne for Diphtheria, Pertusis and Tetanus (DPT)
- Polio Salk vaccine
- Influenza
- Cholera
- Typhus
- Typhoid or paratyphoid.

Deferral of *two weeks* is recommended after the following vaccinations:

- Polio Sabin vaccine (oral)
- Measles
- Mumps
- Yellow fever.

Deferral of *four weeks* is recommended after the following innoculations:

- German measles (Rubella)
- Vaccination by animal serum products like antidiphtheria, anti-venom and anti-gas gangrene.

Deferral should be for *one year* if the vaccination for Rabies is given after the dog bite.

Infectious diseases

The donor suffering from any infectious disease, bacterial or viral is not accepted, so the donors on antibiotics. This is in the interest of the recipient as well as the donor. Though screening of donor's blood for TTDs like: Hepatitis B, Hepatitis C, Syphilis, AIDS and Malaria (In some countries for HTLV1 and 2) are mandatory procedures, but the significance of a proper history cannot be ruled out.

The donor is accepted only, if he does not give a positive history of jaundice in the last one year.

The donor is permanently deferred if his blood has caused hepatitis in the recipient with in six months of transfusion.

Tattooing

The donor who has undergone tattooing on his body in the last six months is deferred.

Malaria

In case of malaria the criteria for deferral is different for endemic and non-endemic areas.

In places like the Indian subcontinent and Saharan African countries where malaria *is endemic*, the blood banks cannot afford to defer a donor on the history of malaria, even in the recent past. Such cases are accepted three months after being cured by antimalarials.

In cases of *non-endemic* areas like USA and Europe, the donor is deferred for three years after a bout of malaria and for six months to one year, if he has visited an endemic area.

Physical examination

Age

The lower age limit of 17-18 years takes account of the high iron requirements of adolescence, and the age of consent. An upper age limit was arbitrarily set at 60 because of increasing incidence of cardiovascular diseases with age, which may make the removal of 350/450 ml of blood dangerous for the health of the donor. No upper age limit is recommended by AABB. First time donors with an age of over 60 years are discouraged, since they have an increased incidence of adverse effects.

Body weight

Body weight depends on the volume of blood to be collected. The donor should not be less than 45 kg, if 350 ml of blood is to be collected. For donation of 450 ml of blood, the ideal body weight should be more than 50 kg.

Volume

The volume of blood donation should not be more then 13% of the estimated blood volume of the donor in order to protect against vasovagal attacks. The collection bags are designed to contain 350 or 450 ml of blood.

Pulse and blood pressure

The pulse should be regular and the rate should be within 80-100/ minute. The BP should be within 110 to 180 systolic and 70 to 100 diastolic in mm Hg.

Systemic examination

The clinical examination should reveal a normal respiratory, and cardiovascular systems and normally functioning kidneys.

Screening of donor blood

Haemoglobin

The haemoglobin estimation before donation is carried out, usually, by a simple technique based on the specific gravity of a drop of blood introduced into a solution of copper sulphate or by micro haematocrit technique. The acceptable minimum concentrations are 12.5 gm/dl of haemoglobin or 38% of haematocrit.

Blood grouping

Serological tests to ascertain the blood group ABO and Rh are carried out on all blood units. Most centres also test for the Rh C and E antigens. Only donations negative for C, D, and E may be labeled Rh negative. Those tested only for the D antigen and found negative should be labeled Rh(D) negative.

Tests for agents of transfusion transmitted diseases

The greatest concern for any blood bank is transfusion transmitted diseases. Safe blood transfusion and safety of the recipient is the prime concern of transfusion services. The tests to screen the donor's blood for TTD must be carried out. Some of the tests are mandatory all over the world. Few other tests are dependent on local legal systems of the particular country or on the condition of the patient.

The mandatory tests are:

- HBsAg for Hepatitis B
- Anti HCV for Hepatitis C
- Antibodies to HIV1and 2 for AIDS
- VDRL or TPHA or RPR for syphilis
- Peripheral blood examination for malarial parasite.

The optional tests are:

- Anti-HBc (core antibody) in addition to HbsAg
- Antibodies to HTLV1 for adult T cell leukemia lymphoma (ATLL)
- Antibodies to CMV for transfusion to immunocompromised patients.

Screening of donor's blood for antibodies to red cell antigens is designed to pick up antibodies that are clinically important. The donations found to have high antibody titre should not be used.

Testing of group O serum for high titre haemolytic anti-A and anti-B is carried out at some centres, where specific blood group is not available for whole blood transfusion. The practice of substituting specific blood group with O blood should not be allowed to override the principle that a patient should receive the blood of his own group only. The group O blood should not be given to the patients of other groups except in an emergency.

Typing for histocompatibility locus antigens (HLA) is carried out on selected donors as the demand for HLA matched platelets escalates. Such platelets would be used in the treatment of a haemorrhagic, thrombocytopenic patient, who, because of many exposures to blood components, has developed multispecific antibodies to the HLA series of antigens and has become refractory to random platelet treatment.

Frequency of donation

The frequency of donation is normally two or three times a year or at an interval of at least 3 months between two donations, the time by which the iron stores of the body are replenished. The latest recommendation of Red Cross Society of USA is an interval of only 56 days for donation of whole blood.

Collection of blood

The blood should be collected by trained phlebotomists under the supervision of a physician.

Bleeding room

The bleeding room where the donor's blood is collected must be air conditioned and properly ventilated. A television set can also be installed. It would help in reducing the stress and anxiety level, specially in the first time donors.

Specially designed donor couches are available which are electrically operated, where, in case of donor reaction, the foot end can be elevated.

The bleeding room should be equipped with the following emergency kit:

- Liquid ammonia or ammonia capsules
- Disposable syringes 2 ml and 5 ml
- Intravenous infusion (IV) sets
- IV fluids
- Oropharyngeal airway
- Oxygen and mask
- Icepacks (in freezer)
- Tongue blades
- Paper bags for breathing
- Injections; antiemetic, adrenalin, dexamethsone, calcium gluconate and sodium phosphate, etc.

Materials required for phlebotomy

Blood collection bags, which are available as single, double triple or quadruple bags. The choice of the bag depends on the type of the component to be prepared. The bags are supplied in 350 ml and 450 ml capacities containing CPD-A1 or CPD SAG/SAGM anticoagulants. 350 ml bag contains 49 ml, and 450 ml bag 63 ml anticoagulant/ preservative.

- Tourniquet or BP instrument
- Artery forceps, clips
- Rubber ball or wooden bar
- Blood bag weighing balance (automatic machine acting as shaker and balance and equipped with a buzzer is the best option)
- Cotton swabs, methylated spirit and tincture benzoin.

Volume of blood

If the volume of blood collected is less than prescribed for the bag, as usually required in paediatric cases, then the amount of the anticoagulant has to be adjusted accordingly. The formula for adjustment of anticoagulant is:

Amount of anticoagulant withdrawn

$$= 63 \text{ or } 49 - (\text{minus}) \frac{\text{Donor's weight}}{50 \text{ or } 45} \times 63 \text{ or } 49$$

Phlebotomy

Site of venepuncture

The antecubital fossa is the ideal site. The site should be free of any local infection.

- Apply the tourniquet or the BP cuff on the arm about 2-3 inches above the elbow joint, raising the pressure to 50 to 60 mm Hg.
- Ask the donor to close the fist. Select the most prominent, straight and thick vein.
- Clean the area and take all antiseptic measures by applying methylated spirit and tincture of iodine.
- Place the blood bag on a lower plane on the weighing balance and clamp the tube close to the needle.
- Perform the venepuncture in a single clean stroke. Do not mess up with the vein.
- Release the clamp. The blood should start flowing down.
- Ask the donor to keep on pressing the rubber ball.
- The phlebotomist should keep on mixing the anticoagulant and the blood gently if the automatic shaker is not being used.
- If the automatic balancing machine is not in use then the blood collected should be weighed. 367 gm for 350 ml and 472 gm for 450 ml of blood is collected, excluding the weight of the bag and anticoagulant.
- As soon as the required amount of blood is collected, apply a clamp on the tube. Release the tourniquet and after putting a sterile cotton swab on the venepuncture site gently withdraw the needle.
- The segments of the tube attached to the bag are used as pilot samples.
- The blood is pushed back in the tube by compressing the bag and knots are applied or the tube is sealed by electric sealer at few places.
- The needle is detached and destroyed by the needle cutter.
- Keep the blood bag at 4-6°C in the refrigerator. If platelets are to be harvested then at room temperature (20-25°C).

- Seal the venepuncture site by applying tincture benzoin.
- Let the donor remain on the couch for at least 10 minutes.
- The donor should be offered refreshment preferably juices, and should be thanked for donation.
- Throughout this process and until the donor leaves the blood bank, he should never be left unattended.

Instructions to donor after donation of blood

- Drink plenty of fluids; like juices, soft drinks and coffee in the next 24 hours.
- Avoid strenuous exercise, prolonged standing and long self automobile drives or bicycling.
- If bleeding occurs from the venepuncture site, compress and raise the arm.
- Remove the band-aid after 4 hours.
- If there are any signs of fainting, consult a doctor or return to the blood bank.

Complications of blood donation (donor reactions)

However, most of the donors leave the blood bank hail and hearty but a few may develop donor reactions, which can be mild, moderate or severe. But, all types of reactions are manageable. The blood bank personnel must be well trained to identify the signs and symptoms of the reactions and their management. Extracare must be taken in case of first time donors. The adverse donor reactions may be of the following types:

The commonest reaction is vasovagal syndrome, resulting in syncope. The features are:

- Excessive sweating
- Weakness
- Dizziness
- Cold and clammy skin
- Low volume pulse and low BP
- Fainting.

The other common adverse reactions are:

- Nausea and vomiting
- Tetany like symptoms due to hyperventilation. The anxious donor looses an excess of carbon dioxide

- Convulsions
- Haematoma.

Management of donor reactions

The adverse reactions are to be managed on the following lines:

- Stop the bleeding process at the first sign of reaction.
- Release the tourniquet and withdraw the needle.
- Raise the foot end above the level of head.
- Open up donor's collar buttons, loosen tight clothing.
- Apply the cotton soaked in liquid ammonia or crushed ammonia capsule near the nostrils.
- Apply cold compresses (icepacks) on the donor's head.
- Ask the donor to breath in the paper bag, so that he can reinhale the carbon dioxide.
- If the donor vomits, provide him towel or a pan. Tilt his head to a side to avoid aspiration of vomits.
- If convulsions are observed, ensure proper airway. Place a tongue blade between the teeth to prevent tongue bite.
- Monitor the pulse, BP and respiration.
- In case a haematoma develops at the site of venepuncture, place few sterile gauze pieces and press for 10 minutes. Application of ice for few minutes also helps.

Storage and preservation of blood and its components

chapter 11

The first authentic blood preservative was developed by two English scientists, Loutit and Mollison in the year 1943 and it was known as "Acid Citrate Dextrose (ACD)". With the advent of time, much better preservatives have been introduced, in which the normal physiology of the blood is maintained and preservative can be stored for a longer period.

Biochemical changes in the stored blood

RBC

The viability of the red cells depend on the 2-3-DPG and ATP levels. The 2-3-DPG level falls more rapidly than the ATP in the stored blood. The oxygen releasing capacity of the haemoglobin is directly proportional to the 2-3-DPG level. If the 2-3-DPG level falls, less oxygen is released to the tissues. The fall in pH of stored blood also affects 2-3-DPG level.

The other changes which take place in RBC are:

- RBC changes its shape from discoid to spherical
- Osmotic fragility is increased
- There is loss of red cell membrane lipids.

WBC

The wbc become nonfunctional after 24 hours of storage, but they retain their antigenic properties and are quite capable of causing non-haemolytic febrile transfusion reactions in the recipients.

Platelets

The platelets stored at 4-6°C lose their haemostatic properties within 48 hours.

Coagulation factors

The coagulation factors, mainly, V and VIII lose their activity within 72 hours of storage.

Electrolytes

The most important biochemical change in the stored blood is the loss of potassium from the red cells and the intake of sodium from plasma.

The choice of the preservative depends on the percentage of "post-transfusion survival of red cells" and its storage period. Higher the post transfusion survival and longer the storage period, better the preservative.

Preservative solutions

Acid citrate dextrose (ACD)

The ACD is hardly used as a blood preservative anymore in any modern setup, because of its shorter storage time (21 days) and poor viability of cells (70%). It was used with the glass bottles.

Citrate phosphate dextrose (CPD)

It was discovered by Gibson, et al that addition of phosphate in the ACD anticoagulant increases the post-transfusion survival of cells to 80% compared to ACDs 70% after 21 days of storage.

The composition of CPD solution is given below:

- Trisodium citrate (dihydrate) 26.30 gm
- Sodium dihydrogen phosphate 2.28 gm
- Dextrose 25.50 gm
- Citric acid 3.27 gm
- Distilled water 1.0 L

The pH of the solution is 5.6-5.8.

The citrate in the solution acts as the anticoagulant (0.2%) citrate can prevent clotting of 2.5 litres of blood.

Phosphate helps in maintaining the pH of the blood.

Dextrose provides nourishment to the cells and helps in the synthesis of ATP. The post-transfusion survival of cells depend on ATPs.

Citrate phosphate dextrose-adenine (CPDA-1)

It was observed by Simon in 1962 that addition of adenine to the CPD solution increases the post-transfusion survival of cells to 80% and the storage period to 35 *days*. The ATP concentration is higher and the viability is more in adenine blood.

The composition of CPDA -1 is given below:

- Trisodium citrate (dihydrate) 26.30 gm
- Sodium dihydrogen phosphate 2.22 gm

- Dextrose (monohydrate) 31.8 gm
- Adenine 0.275 gm
- Citric acid 3.27 gm
- Distilled water 1 L

The ratio of preservative to blood is 14 ml of CPDA-1 solution for 100 ml of blood. The amount of preservative present in 350 ml and 450 ml capacity bags is 49 ml and 63 ml respectively.

The other preservative CPDA-2 in which the amount of dextrose is increased to 44.6 gm, improves the viability of cells further.

Additive solutions

The commonly used additive solutions are CPD-SAG, CPD-SAGM and CPD-Adsol.

CPD-SAGM

The SAGM stands for Saline-Adenine-Glucose-Mannitol. The four bag system introduced by Hogman, et al in 1978, contains preservative solution in two bags. The bag 1 contains 63 ml of CPD solution while the bag 2 contains 100 ml of SAGM solution.

The composition of the SAGM is as follows:

- Sodium chloride 8.77 gm
- Adenine 0.16 gm
- Glucose 8.99 gm
- Mannitol 5.25 gm
- Distilled water 1 L

450 ml of blood is collected in the primary bag containing CPD solution, the plasma is expressed after centrifugation to the empty bag and then the 100 ml of the SAGM solution is expressed in the primary bag containing red cells. The red cells can be stored for 42 days in SAGM. The post-transfusion survival of cells in SAGM is more than 80%.

CPD-Adsol

The composition of CPD-Adsol is the same as of CPD-SAGM, except that, it contains higher concentrations of glucose, adenine and mannitol, which improves viability of cells considerably.

Long-term storage of red cells

The red cells in frozen state can be stored for years. Freezing damages red cells by intracellular ice formations and hypertonicity. This can be prevented by addition of glycerol. The glycerol limits the ice formation and provides liquid phase for cooling of salts, by permeating the red cells easily during freezing.

Glycerolisation

High glycerol solution

40% w/v concentration of glycerol is known as high glycerol solution. The composition of this solution is as follows (6.2 M glycerol solution):

- 57 gm% of glycerol
- 1.6 gm% Na lactate
- 0.03 gm% KCl
- 25 mEq/L of monobasic and disodium phosphate
- pH 6.8

The red cells are frozen at –180°C over a period of 30 minutes by mechanical refrigeration and then stored at –40 to –50°C for 3 years.

Low glycerol solution

The 20% w/v concentration of glycerol is known as low glycerol solution.

The following is the composition of low glycerol solution:

- 35 gm% of glycerol
- 2.88% of mannitol
- 0.65 gm of sodium chloride.

The red cells are frozen at –190°C using liquid nitrogen for 2-3 minutes and then stored in the gas phase of liquid nitrogen for *3 years*.

Thawing and deglycerolisation

Since the red cells are stored in frozen state, so, they must be brought to body temperature. The process is carried out by keeping the frozen red cells in a water bath at 37°C for 10 minutes. The procedure is known as Thawing.

The glycerol must be removed properly. The principle of deglycerolisation is that frozen red cells are kept first in hypertonic solution, and then moved to less hypertonic and finally to isotonic solution.

Procedure for deglycerolisation

- The 40% w/v glycerolised red cells are diluted in 12% sodium chloride buffered to pH 7.2 with 0.15% disodium phosphate and equilibrated for 5 minutes.

- Wash the red cells in 2 litres of 1.6 % of sodium chloride solution buffered to pH 7.2 with 0.03 gm% of disodium phosphate.
- Finally wash the red cells in isotonic glucose solution, which is prepared in 1 litre of 0.9 gm% of sodium chloride solution, containing 0.2 gm% of glucose buffered with 0.0 65 gm% disodium phosphate to a pH of 6.8.

  The shelf life of deglycerolised blood is *24 hours.*

Indications for long-term storage of RBC in frozen state

- Storage of blood for patients with antibodies against high frequency antigens
- The rare blood groups (e.g. Bombay) can be stored in referral hospitals and regional blood banks
- Storage of autologous blood in patients of rare blood group
- The blood in frozen state is also stored for transfusion to patients already sensitised to leucocyte, platelet antigens or plasma proteins.

Storage of plasma

The fresh frozen plasma (FFP) is stored at *-30°C for 1 year.*

Storage of platelets

The platelets are stored at room temperature (RT) 20-25°C *for 5 days* only. More than 5 days of storage of platelets at RT increases the chance of bacterial contamination of platelets.

The preparation and usage of components is given in detail in chapter on "Blood Components".

chapter 12

Haemolytic disease of the newborn

Haemolytic disease of the newborn (HDN) is a unique autoimmune disease. It is characterized by red cell destruction during foetal life and is caused by a foetomaternal blood group incompatibility.

Aetiopathogenesis

HDN occurs due to blood group incompatibility between mother and foetus. The alloimmunisation in mother occurs mostly at the time of labour as a result of transplacental haemorrhage, or by transfusion of incompatible blood. The IgM antibodies do not cross the placental barrier, but the IgG produced because of immunization of maternal red cells, cross the placenta and haemolyse the fetal red cells leading to HDN.

The following conditions are a must for HDN to occur:

- The woman must be exposed through either pregnancy or trans-fusion to the antigen that she lacks.
- The antigenic exposure must result in immunisation and production of antibody.
- The antibody must have the ability to cross the placental barrier and should have a high titre.
- The fetus must possess the antigen corresponding to the maternal antibody.

During the first pregnancy, no incompatibility exists and the first newborn is unaffected, unless the woman was already sensitised by a previous incompatible blood transfusion.

At birth, red cells from the foetus enter the maternal circulation as the placenta separates from the uterus. These antigenic red cells stimulate the maternal immune system to produce the specific antibody. During subsequent pregnancies with incompatible foetus the antibody crosses the placenta and reacts with the foetal red cells resulting in its destruction.

The ABO, Rh or other blood group incompatibility may lead to HDN.

ABO HDN

ABO HDN is more common than Rh HDN, but the disease appears in milder form compared to Rh HDN. ABO HDN is usually found in O group mothers carrying A or B fetus. The anti-A or anti-B produced in O group mothers is IgG in nature that crosses the placental barrier, but since the A and B antigens are not fully developed in the fetus, the damage is minimised.

How to proceed to *diagnose* ABO HDN?

- DAT on the newborn's blood is usually negative or weakly positive.
- Confirm the presence of anti-A and anti-B in the serum of the mother by excluding antibodies to other blood group antigens through a panel of reagent cells.
- Measure the titre of the anti-A or anti-B antibody in the mothers plasma. A titre higher than 1:32 is significant.
- The cord blood haemoglobin level of the baby is reduced.
- Serum bilirubin level of the newborn is moderately raised and can be controlled by phototherapy.
- Spherocytes are seen in the peripheral blood smear of the newborn.
- The RBC of the newborn show increased osmotic fragility.

Rh HDN

The Rh HDN is not as common as ABO HDN but much severe forms are observed in Rh HDN. The isoimmunisation of Rh negative mothers result from Rh positive pregnancy or prior Rh positive blood transfusion.

At the time of labour transplacental haemorrhage is not uncommon. The Rh positive fetal blood enters the maternal circulation leading to production of anti-D antibodies in 5-10% of Rh negative mothers. Subsequently in the second pregnancy, and as a result of exposure to the Rh (D) positive RBC, the already present anti-D crosses the placental barrier and haemolyse the foetal red cells. This happens only if the anti-D is of high titre.

Rh HDN due to blood transfusion

If the Rh negative mother has already been sensitized by an earlier Rh positive blood transfusion, then the chances of developing HDN in the very first pregnancy are high.

Investigations on newborn

After removing the umbilical cord the blood should be collected from the maternal side of the cord. The blood samples should be collected in two vials, EDTA and plain.

The EDTA vial is to be sent for the following investigations:

- Hb estimation
- ABO grouping

- Rh grouping
- DAT.

The tests done on the plain vial samples are:

- Cord blood bilirubin.
- Detection of alloantibodies in the cord serum.

Antenatal management of Rh (D) negative mother

The purpose of monitoring the Rh D negative mothers is to identify the high risk candidates, and take all necessary precautions to avoid HDN and its worst form; the kernicterus.

The investigations if started earlier the better, but preferably in the 12th week of pregnancy.

The investigations should start in the following order:

- Obstetric history.
- History of previous blood transfusions.
- Antibody screening for Anti-D and for clinically significant IgG antibodies of other blood group systems.
- Titration of antibodies every month. *A titre of* 1: 32 is considered significant and is an indication for amniocentesis.
- Determine father's phenotype with anti-D,-C,-E,-c,-e

Amniocentesis

The amniocentesis is usually carried out after 28th week of gestation. The amniotic fluid is tested for bilirubin levels. If high level of bilirubin is observed, intrauterine transfusion is considered.

Considering the mother's previous medical history, titre of anti-D, level of bilirubin in the amniotic fluid, the following modalities are available:

- Intrauterine transfusion.
- Intraperitonial transfusion.
- Plasmapheresis.
- Premature induction of labour.
- Exchange transfusion in the newborn.

Rh immune globulin

The risk of immunisation decreases to almost 1% if Rh immune globulin (RhIg) is administered postpartum. The risk is further minimised to 0.1% when RhIg is given antepartum at 28 weeks of gestation.

chapter 13

Autoimmune haemolytic anaemia

The autoimmune haemolytic anaemia (AIHA) is defined as a shortened red cell survival mediated through immune response by autoimmune humoral antibodies.

Antibodies that are directed against the individual's own red cells are called autoantibodies.

Most of these antibodies react against high incidence antigens.

There are mainly two types of autoimmune haemolytic anaemias (AIHA).

Warm autoimmune haemolytic anaemia

The warm type of AIHA itself may be of the following varieties:

Idiopathic

Without any demonstrable cause.

Secondary

Secondary to some of the following diseases:

- Lymphoma
- Chronic lymphocytic leukaemia (CLL)
- Systemic lupus erythrematosus (SLE)

The AIHA is usually detected first in the blood bank. The warm AIHA is due to antibodies of IgG or complement class, reacting at 37°C against the own red cell antigens. The commonly seen antibodies are of Rh system, and occasionally, of other blood group system.

The patient presents with a mild anaemia of insidious onset.

The DAT is positive.

Cold autoimmune haemolytic anaemia (cold agglutinin syndrome)

This is also of two types.

Idiopathic

Without any demonstrable cause.

Secondary

This type of AIHA is secondary to the following infections:

- Infectious mononucleosis
- Viral infections
- Mycoplasma pneumoniae infection.

This type of anaemia is due to IgM antibodies reacting at RT (20-24°C). Commonly seen antibody is anti-I.

The anaemia gets worse in winters and the patient may present with haemoglobinuria.

The DAT is positive.

Paroxysmal cold haemoglobinuria (PCH)

This type of AIHA may also be idiopathic or secondary in nature.

The antibody usually responsible for PCH is anti-P.

Drug-induced AIHA

The certain drugs may cause AIHA. Methyldopa is notorious for causing AIHA.

Transfusion in AIHA

It is a hard task to find suitable blood for a patient of AIHA. The blood transfusion should be avoided as far as possible.

The antibody coated on the surface of the RBC can be removed by adsorption or elution techniques.

Xylene elution technique

Materials required are:

- Reagent grade xylene
- 2 ml of properly washed and packed RBC
- Supernatant saline from the last wash.

Procedure

- Mix equal volumes of RBC and normal saline.
- Cover the tube with paraffin film, or stopper cork, and agitate the tube vigorously for 1-2 minutes. Remove the paraffin film.
- Place the tube at 56° C for 10 minutes. Stir the contents of the tube by applicator or shake it gently.
- Centrifuge the tube at 1000 g for 10 minutes.
- Carefully remove and discard the upper layer of xylene and stroma by vacuum application. If stroma is mixed with the xylene, repeat step 4.

- Transfer the eluate into a clean tube and test in parallel with the last wash supernatant.
- Add 2 drops of 30% albumin to the test to prevent the haemolysis by residual xylene.

The eluted antibody is identified by the panel of reagent cells.

When antibody has been identified, the blood free from the corresponding antigen is found for transfusion.

Cold acid elution technique

Materials

- Glycene (0.1 M, pH 3.0) prepared by dissolving 3.75 g of glycene and 2.99 g of sodium chloride in 500 ml of DW. Adjust pH to 3.0 with 12 N HCl. Store at 4°C.
- Phosphate buffer (0.8 M, pH 8.2).
- Chilled isotonic saline at 4°C.
- 1 ml of packed RBC, washed six times.
- Supernatant saline from last wash.

Procedure

- Add 1 ml of chilled saline and 2 ml of glycene to 1 ml of washed packed RBC.
- Mix and incubate the tube in an ice bath for one minute.
- Centrifuge the tube at 1000 g for 2 minutes.
- Transfer the supernatant eluate into a clean test tube, and add 0.1 ml of pH 8.2 phosphate buffer for each 1 ml of eluate.
- Mix and centrifuge at 1000 g for 2 minutes.
- Transfer the supernatant eluate into a clean tube and test in parallel with the final wash supernatant.

Note

- Keep glycene at 4°C during use, to maintain correct pH.
- Phosphate buffer will crystallise on storage at 4°C, redissolve at 37°C before use.

chapter 14

Blood components

The era of whole blood is over, and the components have taken its place. The concept is, when a single unit of whole blood can benefit many patients, why waste it on one patient and transfuse him the components, which he does not require at all.

The introduction of integrated plastic blood bags and the refri-gerated centrifuge in the blood banking has completely revolutionised the transfusion therapy.

The following components can be separated from a single unit of 450 ml blood:

- Red cell concentrate (Packed red cells)
- Platelet concentrates
- Fresh frozen plasma (FFP)
- Cryoprecipitate
- Leucocyte depleted RBC concentrate
- Granulocyte concentrate
- Single donor plasma
- Fibrinogen concentrate
- Factor VIII concentrate.

Preparation of RBC concentrate

The RBC concentrate has a haematocrit of almost 80-95%. The following procedure is applied for preparation of RBC concentrate.

Centrifugation method

- Collect blood preferably in a 450 ml of double or triple bag system.
- The blood bags are kept tightly packed and balanced in the buckets of the refrigerated centrifuge.
- Centrifuge at 5000 g for 5 minutes at 4-6° C.
- Express almost 3/4th of plasma in the satellite bag.
- Seal the tube in between, connecting the two bags.
- Detach the satellite bag
- Keep the bag with red cells at 4-6° C
- Store the plasma bag at – 30° C
- The shelf life of the RBC concentrate is the same as that of whole blood, depending on the preservative used.

Leucocytes depleted red cell concentrate

Leucocyte induced non-haemolytic febrile reactions can be minimised by reducing the number of leucocytes to 0.5×10^9 in the RBC concentrate.

The methods for depletion of leucocytes are as follows:

- Removal of buffy coat by centrifugation.
- Washing of red cells
- Spin and filtration
- Freezing and deglycerolisation.

Leucocyte depletion by centrifugation

The procedure is simple and reliable. This could be achieved by two methods.

Upright Spin

- Collect blood in 450 ml blood bags.
- Keep the bags in the bucket of the centrifuge and balance properly.
- Centrifuge at 5000 g for 5 minutes at 4-6° C.
- Express the plasma, buffy coat and approximately 10-20 ml of upper layer of red cells in the satellite bag.
- Seal the connecting tube and separate the bags.

Inverted spin

- Collect blood in 450 ml blood bags.
- Keep the bags in the buckets in inverted position.
- Centrifuge the bags at 5000 g at 4-6° C for 5 minutes.
- Suspend the bag in inverted position at an intravenous fluid stand after opening the seal between primary and satellite bag.
- The leucocyte poor RBC concentrate is collected in the satellite bag leaving approximately 80 ml of plasma mixed with buffy coat and few red cells in the primary bag.
- Separate bags after double sealing the connecting tube.

Preparation of fresh frozen plasma (FFP)

The plasma collected from a single donor or by plasmapheresis and frozen within 4 hours at -70°C is called fresh frozen plasma (FFP).

Procedure

- Collect 450 ml blood in a double or triple bag.

- The collected blood must be stored at 4-6°C for not more than 4 hours prior to centrifugation.
- Centrifuge the bags at 5000 gm for 5 minutes at 4-6°C in a properly packed and balanced position.
- Express 3/4th of the plasma in the satellite bag.
- Seal the tube and detach the plasma containing satellite bag.
- Freeze the plasma at -70° C in a mechanical freezer within 4 hours.
- The ideal volume of FFP is 200- 250 ml.
- Store the plasma in an inverted position at –30°C (stored for 1 year).

Preparation of platelet concentrate (PC)

Like FFP the platelet concentrate can also be prepared from single donor unit or by apheresis.

Procedure

- Collect blood in a 450 ml triple or quadruple bag, after having a clean neat venepuncture.
- There should be a free flow of blood preferably collected within 8 minutes of venepuncture.
- Place the bags in the buckets and balance them properly.
- First centrifuge at 2000 g for 3 minutes (light spin) at 20-24°C to produce platelet rich plasma (PRP).
- Express the PRP in the platelet bag and seal the tube between primary bag and two satellite bags.
- Centrifuge again at 5000 g (heavy spin) for 5 minutes at 20-24°C.
- Express the plasma into the second satellite bag leaving the platelet concentrate in the platelet bag.
- The ideal volume of platelet concentrate is 40-70 ml.
- Store the platelet concentrate at RT (20-24°C) in a shaker or agitator for 5 days only.

Platelet concentrate (PC)

The specifications for an ideal platelet concentrate are as follows (quality control):

Volume	–	40-70 ml
Platelet yield	–	$>5.5 \times 10^{10}$
Leucocytes	–	$< 10^{8}$
RBC	–	< 0.5 ml
pH	–	> 6.0

Note

The donor who has taken Aspirin in the last 3 days must not be accepted as a donor for PC. The platelets become haemostatically ineffective in the presence of circulating salicylic acid in the blood. The acetylation of platelets cyclooxygenase leads to reduced production of throm-boxane A_2.

Cryoprecipitate

This component consists of precipitated plasma proteins, fibrinogen, factor VIII and von Willebrand factor. The cryo is prepared by rapid freezing within 6 hours and then subsequent thawing of the FFP at 1-6°C.

The standard cryo bag should contain at least 80 IU of factor VIII.

Preparation of cryoprecipitate

- Collect 450 ml of blood in a triple integrated bag, and prepare FFP.
- Express the plasma into the satellite bag and clamp the tubing between primary and satellite bag.
- Freeze the plasma, and keep the RBC at 2-6°C.
- Thaw the plasma at 4°C in a shaking waterbath or in a refrigerator at 2-6°C.
- Centrifuge both bags using heavy spin to separate cryoprecipitate from plasma. Open the closure between the primary and satellite bag.
- Express the plasma back into the red cells in the primary container.
- Seal the tubing twice and cut between the seals to separate the two bags.
- Immediately refreeze the cryoprecipitate.
- Keep the whole blood at 2-6°C in the refrigerator.

chapter 15

Transfusion therapy

The whole blood or blood components are used like other pharmacy products to treat and manage patients. The appropriate use of blood and its components is of prime importance for safety of blood transfusion. The guidelines have been laid and certain criteria fixed by the WHO, AABB, American Red Cross Society and National AIDS Control Organisation (NACO) of India for proper usage of blood and its components.

These guidelines have been given as the consensus views of the transfusion medicine specialists in order to minimise the risks of transfusion and to check the misuse of blood and its products. They are not intended to serve as absolute medical indications.

Criteria for whole blood (WB) transfusion

The concept of WB transfusion is obsolete and must be discouraged. There are very few indications of WB transfusion listed below:

- Active bleeding and evidence of blood loss greater than, or equal to 20% of the total blood volume.
- Active bleeding and prior transfusions with two units or more of RBC concentrate (Packed cells).
- Packed cells not available.

Criteria for RBC concentrate transfusion in adults

The major indications are prevention or treatment of symptoms of tissue hypoxia by increasing the oxygen carrying capacity of blood.

Non-surgical cases

- Haemoglobin less than 8 gm/dl.
- Haemoglobin less than 10 gm/dl with severe anaemia symptoms.
- Prophylactic transfusion in patients of anaemia with Hb greater than 8 gm/dl with associated diagnosis of coronary disease, cerebrovascular or chronic pulmonary disease.
- Hb less than 11 gm/dl in a patient who is bleeding and having symptoms of anaemia.

Surgical cases

- Preoperative transfusion is required if the following criteria are met:
  - Hb < 9 gm/dl with impending major blood loss
  - Major or emergency surgery
- Acute blood loss of greater than 500 ml with severe cardiac, vascular or pulmonary disease.
- Acute blood loss greater than 1000 ml with hypotension even after fluid replacement.
- Acute blood loss of 200 ml per hour.

Dosage and administration

The WB and red cells should be ABO and Rh compatible. The RBC concentrate transfusion of one unit in an adult of 70 kg increases the haemoglobin level 1 gm/dl in the absence of continuing blood loss. Transfusion should be completed within 4 hours per unit.

The need for transfusion does not arise with proper diagnosis and treatment of nutritional anaemias.

Criteria for FFP transfusion

The FFP is transfused to correct plasma factor deficiencies. It must never be used to correct hypovolaemia. The choice of fluids for correction of volume is crystalloid and synthetic colloid solutions. The plasma should be thawed before use. The plasma thawed at 30-37°C and maintained at 1-6°C can be stored for 5 days. The thawed plasma is depleted in factor VIII, von Willebrand factor and fibrinogen. It should not be used to treat the patients with deficiency of these factors.

The following criteria are recommended for FFP transfusion in adults:

- Prothrombin Time (PT) and Activated Partial Thromboplastin Time (APTT) more than 1.5 times of the midpoint of the normal values.
- Generalised oozing or uncontrolled intraoperative oozing.
- Massive RBC transfusion of more than 8 units /24 hours.
- Treatment of thrombotic thrombocytopenic purpura (TTP), haemolytic uraemic syndrome.
- Treatment of antithrombin-III deficiency in patients who require heparin and are heparin refractory.
- Replacement during plasma exchange.

Transfusion of cryoprecipitate

The cold insoluble portion of plasma that precipitates when plasma is thawed at 1-6°C is known as cryoprecipitate. This cryoprecipitate is stored at –18°C. Cryoprecipitate provides therapeutic amounts of factor VIII:C, factor XIII, von Willebrand factor and fibrinogen.

Indications for Transfusion of Cryoprecipitate

- Treatment of bleeding due to hypofibrinogenaemia or dys-fibrinogenaemia.
- Treatment of DIC.
- Prophylaxis or treatment of Haemophilia A (deficiency of factor VIII).

Cryoprecipitate should not be used in the treatment of Haemophilia B/Christmas disease (factor IX deficiency).

Cryoprecipitate is administered after pooling. It should be ABO compatible. Rh type does not matter.

Dosage

Ten bags of fibrinogen increases the fibrinogen level of a 70 kg patient to approximately 70 mg/dl.

Transfusion of platelet concentrate

The platelets concentrate can be produced either manually from a donor or by apheresis. The following types of major platelet products are available.

- *Random donor platelets (RDP):* Collected from a donor and prepared manually.
- *Single donor platelets (SDP):* Harvested from a single donor by apheresis. A single unit of platelet concentrate produced by apheresis is almost equal to 8 units of manually produced RDPs from 8 donors.
- *Pooled platelets:* Prepared from 4-6 units of RDP pooled together.
- Platelet transfusion is recommended in cases of haemorrhagic manifestations either from thrombocytopenia or from functional disorders of platelets.

Criteria for platelet transfusion

The following criteria or tansfusion triggers for platelets are recommended:

- Platelet count less than 10,000/µl, not due to Idiopathic Thrombocytopenic Purpura (ITP), TTP and haemolytic uraemic syndrome.
- Platelet count between 10,000 and 20,000/µl with coagulation abnormalities, or extensive petechiae or ecchymoses.

- Platelet count less than 50,000/µl in a patient who is bleeding.
- Platelet count greater than 1,00,000/µl, requiring red cell transfusion prior to major surgery.
- Platelet count greater than 1,00,000/µl or normal count with one of the following:
  a. Bleeding with platelet dysfunction and a documented pro-longed bleeding time of more than 10 minutes.
  b. Massive RBC transfusion of more than 8 units within 24 hours.
  c. Cardiovascular surgery with RBC transfusion of more than 6 units.

Factors affecting response to platelet transfusion

The following conditions may not give desired results of platelet transfusion:

- Bleeding
- Fever
- Infection
- Splenomegaly
- Disseminated intravascular coagulation (DIC)
- Uraemia
- Antibodies to human platelet antigens (HPA) or human leucocyte antigens (HLA).

Platelet increment

The ideal platelet transfusion provides an increment of 7,500-10,000/µl of platelet count one hour after the transfusion.

ABO compatibility for platelet concentrate (PC) is not necessary, but ABO compatible PC provides higher platelet increments.

One unit of SDP or 4-6 pooled RDPs raise the platelet count of a 70 kg man approximately, 30,000-50,000/µl. Platelet increment may be lower than desired in the presence of fever, splenomegaly, infection, certain medications or alloimmunisation to HLA or HPA.

Requirement of platelets

The transfusion medicine specialist can calculate the dose (No. of units) of the required PC in consultation with the physician.

The number of units of platelets required is calculated from the following formula:

$$N = (P_1 - P_0) \times BSA / 10$$

- N is the number of units required
- P_1 is the desired platelet count
- P_0 is the initial platelet count
- BSA is the body surface area estimated from height and weight.

Platelet refractoriness

It has been observed that most of the patients receiving PC from random donors do not show the desired increment and become refractory or alloimmunised to HLA and HPA.

The refractoriness is defined as the failure of the two consecutive transfusions to give a corrected increment of greater than 7,500/µl, one hour after transfusion of a single unit of RDP, in the absence of fever, infection, haemorrhage, splenomegaly or DIC.

The use of filters for platelet transfusion is recommended. Different types of bed side filters are available for platelet transfusion.

Transfusion of fresh blood

Some physicians appear to be obsessed with "fresh blood transfusion" which carries no definite connotation. Since blood must be screened for HIV and other transfusion transmitted viruses, requiring sufficient time and samples, so, it is not possible to arrange fresh blood in emergency. The fresh blood has no definite advantage when the post- transfusion survival of the stored red cells is as good. There are very few indications for transfusion of fresh blood.

Massive transfusion

The massive blood transfusion is defined as replacement of patient's total blood volume by stored blood in less than 24 hours. The priorities are to maintain haemostasis and metabolic disturbances.

The complications are thrombocytopenia, hyperkalaemia and hypocalcaemia.

Autologous blood transfusion

The autologous blood transfusion is defined as transfusion of patient's own blood. The other routinely practiced transfusion is homologous transfusion.

Even with the mandatory screening for most of the diseases transmitted through blood, the safety of the transfusion is not guaranteed. In view of this, the autologous blood transfusion remains the best bet.

The indications for autologous transfusion are:

- Patients with rare blood group or carrying antibodies against commonly present antigens.
- Patients with Bombay blood group.
- To minimise risk of blood transmitted diseases.

Options for autologous transfusion

Predeposit

The blood is collected weeks before the date of planned surgery and then transfused at the time of operation. This requires proper storage facility. The contraindications are: active bacterial infection and Hb level less than 11 gm/dl.

Normovolumic haemodilution

Preoperative or Intraoperative normovolumic haemodilution is safe. The patients who are not anaemic get almost their quarter volume withdrawn, immediately before operation and replaced by volume expander. The collected blood is transfused after the surgery is over. This prevents the excessive loss of red cells during surgery.

The volume of blood to be collected for a given haematocrit is determined by the following formula:

$$\text{Volume of blood removed} = \frac{\text{Estimated blood volume} \times \text{Initial PCV} - \text{desired PCV}}{\text{Mean of PCV (initial + desired)}}$$

Intraoperative salvage

The cell savers collect the blood lost during surgery and the blood is reinfused after the surgery **(Figure 15.1)**.

Steps of intraoperative blood salvage (Figure 15.2)

Step -1: Suction
Step -2: Collection and filtration
Step -3: Preparation
Step -4: Separation
Step -5: Waste disposal
Step -6: Red cell salvage
Step -7: Re-infusion.

Postoperative salvage

The blood lost through oozing during the postsurgical phase and collected by cell saver is reinfused to the patient.

The salvage procedures have definite advantage where operative losses are very high.

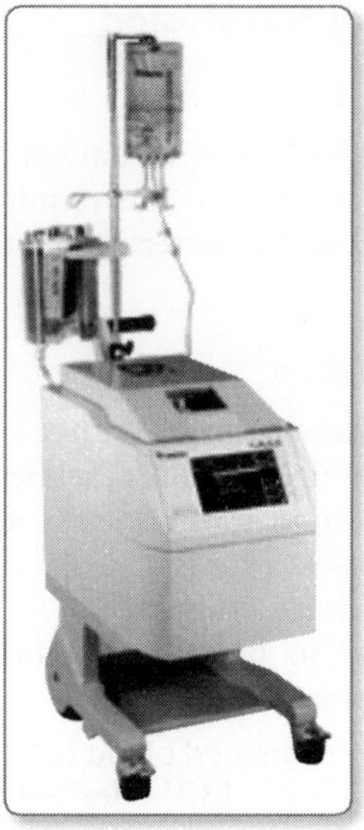

Figure 15.1: Intraoperative blood salvage machine (Cell Saver)
(For colour version, see Plate 4)

Single unit transfusion

The single unit transfusion must be discouraged because they cause more harm than benefit to the patients.

Apheresis/hemapheresis

Apheresis means "to take away". Apheresis is the procedure where desired component is collected from a donor and the unwanted components are returned back to the donor's circulatory system, through apheresis machine known as cell separators **(Figure 15.3)**.

The desired component can be: red cell concentrate, platelets, plasma or granulocytes.

The advantages of apheresis are:

- The donor donates only one component and saves the other
- That increases the frequency of donation of the donor. A platelets donor (SDP) can donate again after 72 hours.
- The yield of the product is very high.

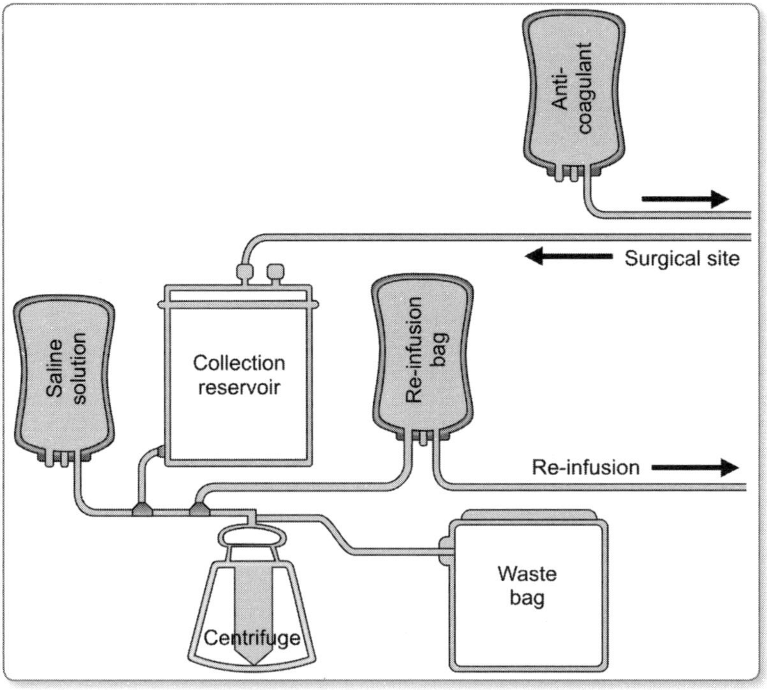

Figure 15.2: Intraoperative blood salvage diagram
(For colour version, see Plate 5)

- The apheresis platelet which is called single donor platelet (SDP) reduces the risk of platelet refractoriness.
- The component is prepared in a much shorter span of time.

Disadvantages

The disadvantages are very few:

- The whole process of Apheresis takes almost 2 hours, which may be longer for the donor, but he can enjoy television watching during the period of donation.
- Occasionally, some donors develop tetany like symptoms due to hypocalcemia caused by calcium consumption by circulating anticoagulants.

Two types of systems of separators are available:

- Intermittent flow separator (IFS)
- Continuous flow separator (CFS).

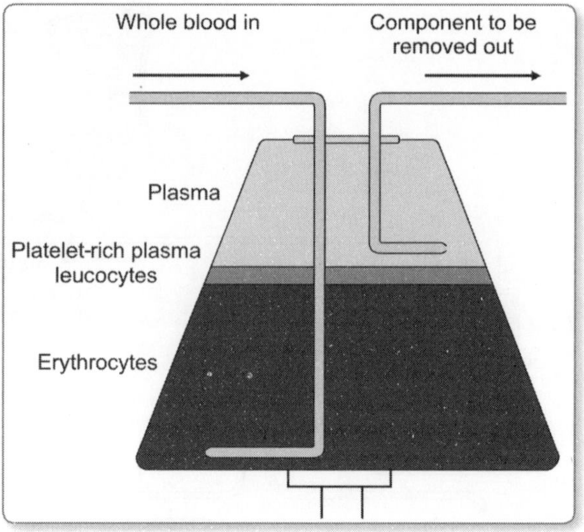

Figure 15.3: Diagrammatic presentation of functioning of apheresis *(For colour version, see Plate 5)*

Both types of separators have their advantages and disadvantages. In the IFS only one intravenous access is required for collection and return which results in longer duration for the whole process. The CFS requires two intravenous accesses **(Figure 15.4)**. The process is faster but the yield is less.

Frequency of donation

- Plasma donors can donate twice a week.
- Platelet donors can donate a maximum of 24 times in a year.

Therapeutic apheresis

Apheresis can be applied for therapeutic purposes too **(Figure 15.5)**.

Indications for therapeutic apheresis

- *Total plasma exchange:* The diseased plasma is completely withdrawn and replaced by fresh healthy plasma.
- *Hyperleucocytosis:* In certain cases of leukemias like; CLL the leucocyte component is withdrawn to reduce the load of hyper-leucocytosis.
- *Essential thrombocythemia:* The platelets counts which may exceed 10 million/µl in essential thrombocythemia may be reduced by extracting platelets.
- Guillian-Barre syndrome

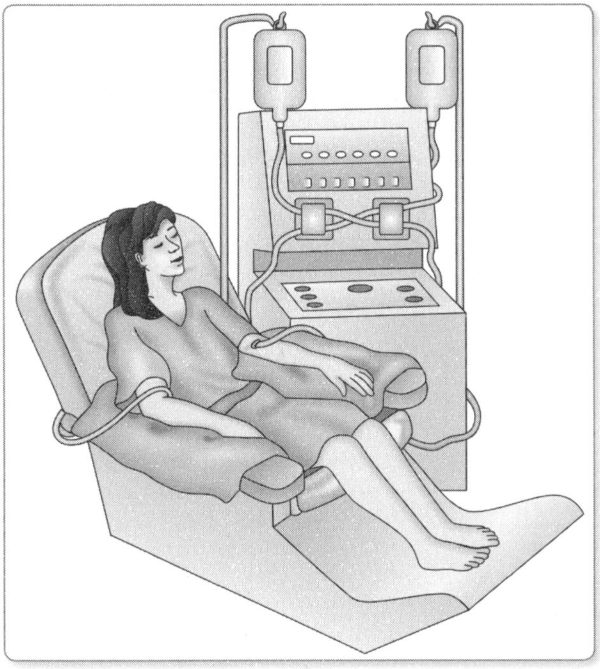

Figure 15.4: Functioning of a continuous flow separator
(For colour version, see Plate 6)

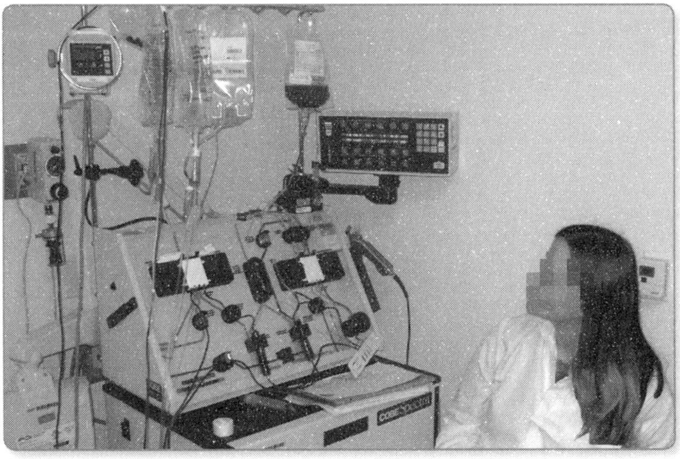

Figure 15.5: Therapeutic apheresis in progress
(For colour version, see Plate 6)

Hospital transfusion committee

It is almost imperative for each hospital to have a hospital transfusion committee (HTC). The committee should comprise of clinicians (Users) specially surgeons, anesthetists, gynaecologists, oncologists, nursing staff and blood transfusion specialists. A clinician should preferably head the committee.

The job of HTC is to formulate policies for proper use of blood and components and monitoring of adverse effects of transfusion.

Neonatal and pediatric transfusion

chapter 16

From birth to four months is known as the neonatal period. Neonates quite often require blood transfusion and their requirements are different and unique. A normal neonate has approximately 85 ml/kg of blood volume. Frequent blood collection for laboratory investigations leads to iatrogenic blood loss and need for transfusion.

Blood grouping of newborns or cord blood

ABO grouping

The ABO antigens are not fully developed on the red cells of a newborn. The naturally occurring complete antibodies are also not present. Whatever alloantibodies are present in the cord blood are of maternal origin. The reverse grouping is not recommended on newborn's blood. The cord blood contains Wharton's jelly, which may lead to error unless the cord cells are thoroughly washed 3-4 times in saline.

Rh grouping

In a normal neonate the routine Rh grouping poses no problem, unless the neonatal red cells are heavily coated by IgG antibodies. The contamination by Wharton's jelly may also lead to inaccurate result. In case of Rh hemolytic disease of newborn (HDN), the neonatal red cells may be fully saturated with maternal anti-D leading to "blocked D". The anti-D reagent may not react with the unavailable antigen leading to a false negative result. The forward ABO blood grouping and Rh-D can also be performed by the gel card technique. The card has 6 microtubes **(Figure 16.1)**.
The sixth microtube carries AHG reagent and used for DAT. The requirements and procedure for the blood grouping and DAT is similar to that employed in cases of adults.

Anti-human globulin (AHG) test (Coombs')

The direct antiglobulin test (DAT) is strongly positive in HDN. If the DAT is positive and the maternal serum is negative for antibody screen, there is a strong possibility of ABO HDN or HDN due to low incidence antigen. In case of low incidence antigen HDN the elute should be tested against the father's red cells. For confirmation, mother's serum against father's cells should be tested.

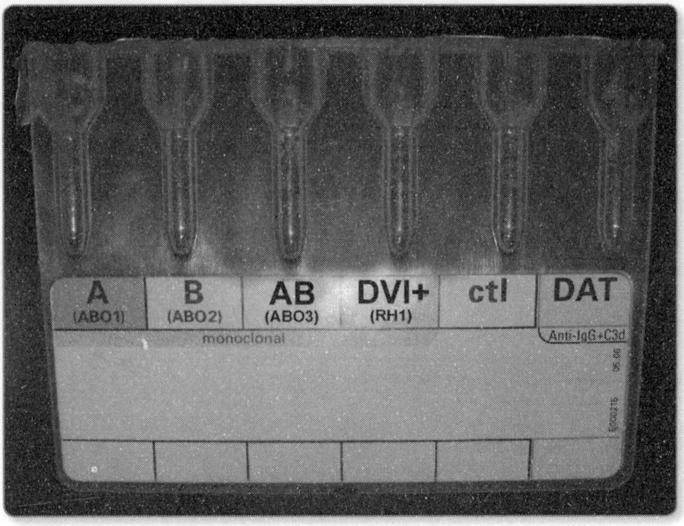

Figure 16.1: ABO blood grouping for newborns and DAT

(For colour version, see Plate 7)

Cross-matching in neonates

If antibody screen is negative and the neonate has been transfused with O negative or ABO compatible blood then compatibility testing can be omitted. If unexpected antibodies are detected in neonate or mother's serum then compatibility testing must be carried out. If the neonate is to receive RBC concentrate of an ABO group incompatible with mother's serum, it is necessary to cross-match the RBC with neonate's serum.

Procedure

- Determine the ABO and Rh(D) grouping of the neonate by forward grouping only.
- Perform DAT on the neonate's red cells for Haemolytic Disease of Newborn (HDN).
- Screen the maternal serum for any alloantibody.
- When DAT on neonate's cells and the IAT on mother's serum are negative, cross-match the group specific donor cells with the neonate's serum.
- If the antibody screening on mother's serum is positive or the DAT on neonate's cells is positive (HDN), the donor's cells must be cross-matched with the maternal serum.

- If group O blood is to be given to group A or B recipient then RBC concentrate and not whole blood is recommended.

Frequent blood sampling, especially for monitoring blood gases may result in requirement for transfusion to replace the blood lost in phlebotomy.

Components transfusion in neonates

Red cells concentrate

The neonates require small amounts of blood transfusion. Many aliquots can be prepared from a single unit of blood or small amount of blood may be collected from a donor after adjusting the blood and anticoagulant ratio. A single unit of blood can provide 12 aliquots of 20 ml each and a unit of FFP. Units containing 30-60 ml of whole blood (WB) can also be collected. A unit intended for WB should be collected in a double bag. The unit intended for component preparation of RBC, FFP and PC should be collected in a set of quadruple bags.

Criteria for RBC concentrate transfusion in neonates

- Hb < 13 gm/dl (Hct < 40 %) with severe cardiopulmonary disease.
- Hb < 10 gm/dl (30 < %) with moderate cardiopulmonary disease.
- Hb < 8 gm /dl (24%) with symptomatic anaemia or surgery.
- Phlebotomy or bleeding exceeding 25% of blood volume.
- 10-20 ml/ kg body wt of RBC transfusion is appropriate.
- RBC concentrate of < 7 day old is required only for large volume of transfusion.

Definitions of severe, moderate, symptomatic must be locally defined. There is no proven benefit of replacing iatrogenic blood loss by volume; instead transfusion should be done to maintain minimum hematocrit.

Criteria for FFP transfusion in neonates

Most infants have low levels of vitamin K dependant factors; hence, all infants receive vitamin K at birth. It has been observed that IM vitamin K is more effective.

Many infants, especially premature normally have prolonged INR. The prolongation of INR, in absence of clinical bleeding or significant risk of bleeding is not an indication for plasma transfusion.

Plasma 10-15 ml/kg is usual dose for infants. Cryoprecipitate may be required if treating fibrinogen level <100.

The criteria for FFP transfusion in neonates are slightly different from adults.

- Reconstitution of RBC concentrates to simulate whole blood for use in exchange transfusion.
- Hemorrhage secondary to vitamin K deficiency.
- Disseminated intravascular coagulation (DIC) with bleeding.
- Bleeding in congenital coagulation factor deficiency.

Platelet transfusion

The underlying maternal conditions like, severe pre-eclampsia, sepsis or Necrotising Enterocolitis (NEC) may lead to thrombocytopenia in neonates.

The randomized trials have shown no benefit of platelet transfusion with a 150000/ul trigger vs 50000 /ul trigger in neonates. Role of prophylactic platelet transfusions is also unproven.

However, general consensus support platelet transfusion for neonates with a platelet count of <50000 /ul with or without clinical signs.

Criteria for platelet transfusion in neonates:

The criteria of platelet transfusion in neonates are not very different from adults. The following criteria are universally accepted:

- Platelets < 100,000/ul and the patient bleeding or clinically unstable.
- Platelets < 50,000/ul and undergoing an invasive procedure.
- Platelets < 20,000/ul and even with no signs of bleeding and clinically stable.
- Volume of 10 ml/kg body wt. is appropriate for transfusion.

Transfusion of platelets in NAIT and NITP

The two conditions Neonatal Alloimmune Thrombocytopenia (NAIT) and Neonatal Autoimmune Thrombocytopenic Purpura (NITP) may lead to thrombocytopenia in neonates d ue to isoimmunisation and maternal alloantibodies. In cases where HPA incompatibility is not known , free of plasma and irradiated maternal platelets is an ideal choice.

Transfusion in preterm neonates

Studies have revealed that a transfusion of 20 ml/kg in preterm babies results in larger rise in hemoglobin levels than a transfusion of smaller amounts of RBC concentrate.

The guidelines for transfusion in cases of preterm neonates vary with the age of the neonate. Twenty eight days of age signifies the transfusion trigger.

Ventilation status	No spontaneous ventilation		Spontaneous ventilation	
Age	<28 days	> 28 days	<28 days	> 28 days
Transfusion trigger	Hb ; 12 gm/dl (Hct; 40%)	Hb;10 gm/dl (Hct; 30%)	Hb;10 gm/dl (Hct; 30%)	Hb; 8 gm/dl (Hct; 25%)

Exchange blood transfusion

In exchange transfusion the blood volume is replaced by fresh blood. This is one genuine reason for use of fresh blood, where blood not more than 5 days old is recommended.

The indications for exchange transfusion are:

- Haemolytic disease of newborn (HDN)
- Sickle cell anaemia
- Severe neonatal sepsis
- Life-threatening hyperkalemia
- Drug toxicity

Exchange transfusion should be done before serum bilirubin of the neonate rises to the levels at which CNS damage occurs due to kernicterus.

Cross-matching for exchange transfusion

The serum or plasma of either mother or neonate can be used for cross-matching with the donor's RBC. Transfused blood should be of the same ABO and Rh group as of neonate. If blood is cross-matched against mother's serum, it should be O Rh negative. An exchange transfusion equal to twice the newborn's blood volume is recommended. The blood volume of a full term newborn is approximately 85 ml/kg of body weight. Volume of whole blood required for two volume exchange transfusion is calculated as:

Weight of newborn in kg × 85 × 2

Two catheters of identical size are required for isovolumetric method. The umbilical artery is used for withdrawal and umbilical vein for infusion.

A maximum of 5 ml/kg is used for each withdrawal and infusion every three minutes.

Complications of exchange transfusion

The following complications are observed in exchange transfusion:

- Hypoglycaemia
- Hypovolaemia

- Hypocalcaemia
- Thrombocytopenia.

Intrauterine transfusion

Intrauterine transfusion can be performed after 24th week of gestation. The procedure is performed under radiographic monitoring. A needle is passed through the mother's abdomen and uterine wall into the fetal abdominal cavity. The transfused red cells enter the fetal circulation by absorption from the lymphatic channels. An intrauterine exchange transfusion, under ultrasound guidance can also be performed through the umbilical vein.

The high level of bile pigments in the amniotic fluid, a sign of fetal haemolysis in cases of impending HDN, is an indication for intrauterine transfusion.

The blood for intrauterine transfusion should be as fresh as possible. Blood should be cross-matched with the mother's serum. The packed RBC should have a hematocrit of 80-85 %. The blood should be leukodepleted and irradiated.

Cytomegalovirus infection

Cytomegalovirus (CMV) infection may occur in perinatal period or can be harboured from mother's breast feed or nursery personnel. CMV is also transmitted by blood transfusion which can be and should be avoided. The CMV is carried by leukocytes. The premature and under weight babies requiring multiple transfusions are at a higher risk of CMV infection.

The washing of red cells and leukocyte depleted red cells diminish the chances of acquired CMV infection.

chapter 17

Obstetrical transfusion practice

Massive perioperative or periparturitional bleeding occasionally occurs in obstetric and gynaecologic patients. Placenta previa, uterine atony, ectopic pregnancy and postpartum haemorrhage are just a few examples of many conditions that could predispose patients to significant blood loss. Therefore, it is important for obstetricians and gynaecologists to be proficient in managing episodes of massive haemorrhage and the practice of most commonly used blood components. Postpartum haemorrhage (PPH) is one of the top 5 causes of maternal mortality in developed and developing countries. The incidence of PPH is 40% after vaginal delivery and 30% after cesarean section. Criteria for transfusion in PPH are based on the amount of blood lost. In clinical obstetrics, exact measurement of blood loss is often difficult. The most important treatment of PPH is red cell concentrate transfusion. In the past few years, increasing concern has arisen about this treatment. Despite the introduction of several new guidelines, transfusion criteria still vary widely between clinicians. The decision whether to prescribe RBC transfusion, is mostly based on postpartum hemoglobin (Hb) values. RBC transfusion should be aimed to reduce morbidity.

Criteria for obstetric transfusion

The aim of these guidelines is to offer guidance about the appropriate use of blood in obstetric cases as well as to minimise blood loss. Active management of third stage of labour is crucial in minimising the blood loss.

Anaemia in pregnancy

Anaemia should be treated first. If the haemoglobin level is less than 10.5 gm/dl in the antennal period, iron deficiency anaemia should be considered, once the haemoglobinopathies have been ruled out. Oral iron therapy is recommended. Parenteral iron therapy should be considered only when oral iron is not tolerated or absorbed.

Anaemia of hemoglobinopathies has to be managed by blood transfusions.

Antenatal care

All pregnant women should have their blood group and antibodies status checked at 28 weeks of gestation. In known cases of Rh negative mothers pregnant with Rh positive fetus, regular monitoring of anti-D titre should be carried out in the second and subsequent pregnancies. An anti-D titre of > 1:32 is a sign of impending HDN and requires special precautions for the pregnant woman and fetus.

Transfusion therapy in obstetrics

- Patient blood samples used for crossmatching should be no more than 7 days old.
- The decision to perform transfusion should be based on haematological and clinical profile of patient. Transfusion is rarely indicated in a stable patient with Hb greater than 10 gm/ dl. Transfusion is almost always indicated when Hb level is less than 6 gm/dl.
- Preferably, a Kell- negative blood should be used for transfusion to avoid HDN.
- The safer trigger for transfusion of platelets in a profusely bleeding patient is 75000/μl of platelets. The platelet count should be maintained at >50000/ μl. The recommendation of Indian Society of Hematology and Transfusion (ISHBT) for platelet threshold for vaginal delivery is 30000/ μl, for cesarean section is 50000/ μl and for epidural anesthesia is 80000/ μl.
- The red cells and platelets concentrate for transfusion should be preferably CMV seronegative, however, urgent transfusions are not delayed if CMV negative blood is not available.
- The platelet, FFP and cryoprecipitate ideally should be of the same ABO group as of the recipient.
- RhD negative women should be given RhD negative platelets, otherwise in case of transfusion of Rh D positive platelets they require anti-Rh D immunoglobulin in a dose of 250 IU.
- Predeposit autologous transfusion is not an option in pregnancy.
- Blood salvage is recommended in patients where intraoperative blood loss is expected to be greater than 1500 ml.

Transfusion in DIC

Obstetric conditions predisposing to DIC include amniotic fluid embolism, placenta abruption and pre-eclampsia. DIC is known as consumption coagulopathy presenting with hypofibrinogenemia, coagulation factor deficiency and thrombocytopenia. Pregnant women have higher fibrinogen levels than non-pregnant women and should be considered severely hypofibrinogenaemic when the fibrinogen level is <1.5 g/L.

DIC is suspected if the patient has got the following hematological profile:

- Platelet count < 50000 / µl.
- PT and PTT > 1.5 times of normal range
- INR > 1.5
- Fibrinogen < 1.0 g/L

In cases of DIC or a total blood loss of almost 1 volume of blood, a combination of platelets, FFP and cryoprecipitate is recommended. Fibrinogen level should be maintained above 1.0 gm/L.

- Platelet transfusion to maintain a platelet count at >50000 / µl.
- FFP 12-15 ml/kg of body wt is given to keep the PTT/aPTT and PT ratios at less than 1:5 times of normal
- Cryoprecipitate is the appropriate choice for hypofibrinogenaemia.

Massive transfusion

Massive blood loss may be defined as the loss of 1 blood volume within a 24-hour period. Normal blood volume in the adult is taken as approximately 7% of ideal body weight. Other definitions include 50% blood volume loss within 3 hours or a rate of loss of 150 ml/minute.

Postpartum hemorrhage and ectopic pregnancy are very common causes of massive blood loss which may require massive transfusion.

Most of the advanced blood banks have formulated guidelines for initiating a massive transfusion in the name of "Massive Transfusion Protocol" (MTP). When MTP should be activated in case of a severely bleeding patient is guided by the following criteria:

- Patients with estimated blood loss of > 2500 ml.
- Patients who have already received four units of red cell concentrate and transfusion of more units are anticipated.
- Evidence of coagulopathy in a patient.

Further Reading

1. Action Plan for Blood Safety Under NACP-III (2007-2012), NACO, India.
2. Blood Bank Management System—A Monitoring Tool for Blood Bank Standards; Proceedings of ASCNT, CDAC, NOIDA, India, 2011.
3. Blood Safety by World Health Organization; Fact Sheet, June 2011.
4. Guidelines for Setting up of Blood Storage Centres at First Referral Units; Maternal Health Division, Department of Family Welfare, Government of India, 2003.
5. Gundu Rao HR. Handbook of Blood Banking and Transfusion Medicine, Jaypee Brothers Medical Publishers, New Delhi, 2006.
6. Harmening DM. Modern Blood Banking and Transfusion Practices, 6th edn, Textbooks and Handbooks, Philadelphia, FA Davis Company, 2012.
7. Judd WJ. Judd's Method of Immunohematology, 3rd edn, Karger, 2008.
8. Laboratory Manual for Technicians (ICTC, PPTCTC, Blood Banks, PHC), by NACO, India, 2007.
9. Roback JD. AABB Technical Manual , 17th edn, 2011.
10. Rudmann SV. Textbook of Blood Banking and Transfusion Medicine, Elsevier, 2005.

Index

Page numbers followed by *f* refer to figure and *t* refer to table

S

T